Summa Health System
Department
Ophthalmology

Rec'd 2/2/08

DVD - Available in
Dept Oph Office.

D1329767

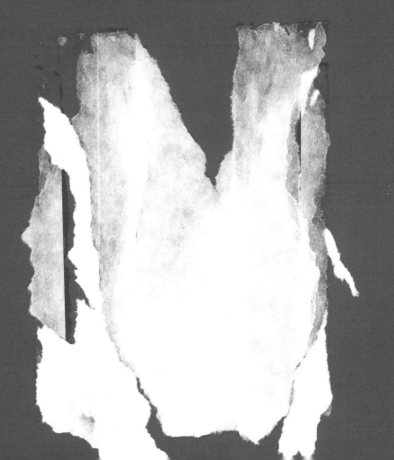

Cataract Surgery

Surgical Techniques in Ophthalmology

Series Editors

F Hampton Roy MD FACS **and Larry Benjamin** FRCS FRCOphth DO

Strabismus Surgery
ISBN 978 1 4160 3020 1

Cataract Surgery
ISBN 978 1 4160 2969 4

Glaucoma Surgery
ISBN 978 1 4160 3021 8

Refractive Surgery
ISBN 978 1 4160 3022 5

Retina and Vitreous Surgery
ISBN 978 1 4160 4206 8

Oculoplastic Surgery
ISBN 978 1 4160 3286 1

Cataract Surgery

Edited by

Larry Benjamin FRCS FRCOphth DO
Consultant Ophthalmic Surgeon
Department of Ophthalmology
Stoke Mandeville Hospital NHS Trust
Aylesbury, UK

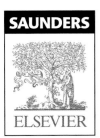

SAUNDERS

ELSEVIER

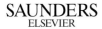

© 2007, Elsevier Inc. All rights reserved.

Chapter 7
© Brian Little, DO FRCS FRCOphth, Consultant Ophthalmologist and
Hon Senior Lecturer, Royal Free Hospital, London, UK.

First published 2007

No part of this publication may be reproduced, stored in a retrieval system,
or transmitted in any form or by any means, electronic, mechanical,
photocopying, recording or otherwise, without the prior permission of the
Publishers. Permissions may be sought directly from Elsevier's Health
Sciences Rights Department, 1600 John F. Kennedy Boulevard, Suite 1800,
Philadelphia, PA 19103-2899, USA: phone: (+1) 215 239 3804; fax:
(+1) 215 239 3805; or, e-mail: *healthpermissions@elsevier.com*. You may
also complete your request on-line via the Elsevier homepage
(http://www.elsevier.com), by selecting 'Support and contact' and then
'Copyright and Permission'.

ISBN 978 1 4160 2969 4

British Library Cataloguing in Publication Data
A catalogue record for this book is available from the British Library

Library of Congress Cataloging in Publication Data
A catalog record for this book is available from the Library of Congress

Notice
Medical knowledge is constantly changing. Standard safety precautions
must be followed, but as new research and clinical experience broaden
our knowledge, changes in treatment and drug therapy may become
necessary or appropriate. Readers are advised to check the most current
product information provided by the manufacturer of each drug to be
administered to verify the recommended dose, the method and duration
of administration, and contraindications. It is the responsibility of the
practitioner, relying on experience and knowledge of the patient, to
determine dosages and the best treatment for each individual patient.
Neither the Publisher nor the author assume any liability for any injury
and/or damage to persons or property arising from this publication.
The Publisher

Printed in China
Last digit is the print number: 9 8 7 6 5 4 3 2 1

Working together to grow
libraries in developing countries

www.elsevier.com | www.bookaid.org | www.sabre.org

ELSEVIER   BOOK AID
International   Sabre Foundation

Commissioning Editor: Russell Gabbedy
Development Editor: Joanne Scott
Project Manager: Rory MacDonald
Design Manager: Jayne Jones
Illustration Manager: Gillian Richards
Illustrator: Jennifer Rose
Marketing Managers: Lisa Damico (USA)/John Canelon (UK)

Contents

Series Preface

Modern Ophthalmic surgery is a combination of dexterity, knowledge, judgement and experience which is gained over many years. Properly applied it can produce results which can be life changing for the patient and tremendously rewarding for the team looking after the patient. Complications arising from the surgery can be just as life altering, more so perhaps than in many other branches of surgery because of the emotive implications of loss of sight.

Training in Ophthalmology is becoming shorter and more intense on both sides of the Atlantic and the trainee surgeon needs clear, structured tuition on which to base their practical surgical experience. Theoretical learning of surgery must always be supported by a positive practical learning environment and this series of books aims to help with the theoretical aspects of techniques but also gives good, practical guidance for the time spent in the operating theatre.

Adaptability is the key to successful surgery. Being able to change a surgical plan part of the way through a procedure, implement that change whilst taking the whole team with you and achieving a good outcome while still making the whole process a positive experience for the patient requires skill and judgement. Learning different approaches to a surgical procedure enables that adaptability whereas a surgeon stuck with a single technique will at some point be unable to complete the operation successfully.

This surgical series is written by an international selection of surgeons with many combined years of surgical practice and teaching. Each volume is written in a clear, structured format with many pictures and diagrams and is also coupled with high quality surgical video footage where these help to illustrate an important surgical concept. Whilst no surgical text can be completely comprehensive, the techniques described in the various volumes are all tried and tested by the authors.

It is hoped that these six volumes will help to enable surgical adaptability.

F Hampton Roy
Larry Benjamin

Preface

Modern cataract surgery looks easy in the hands of an expert. To become expert takes many years which not only involves the development of sound microsurgical skills but also an attitude of mind.

Successful removal of the crystalline lens and its replacement with an artificial one is a procedure with a fascinating history which continues to develop and evolve in many ways. This continuing process of innovation is one of the reasons why ophthalmic surgery remains attractive as a specialty.

This volume, one of six in the new Surgical Techniques in Ophthalmology series from Elsevier, aims not only to guide the reader through the procedure in a logical sequence, but also to discuss the facilities, team working and equipment issues which are so important in delivery of a first rate service for patients suffering from cataract.

In addition to addressing the different techniques and equipment for cataract removal, chapters on difficult cases and management of complications are included.

It is hoped that by reading this book and watching the accompanying videos, the learning time for novice surgeons will be shortened and the flexibility and adaptability of established surgeons will be increased.

Larry Benjamin

Acknowledgements

I would like to thank all those at Elsevier who have given support and encouragement in the preparation of this book. Thanks also to Janet Sear for typing the manuscript so expertly and to all my residents, past and present, who bring variety and stimulation to my job as a surgeon and as a trainer, both of which I regard as a privilege.

Finally, I would like to thank my family Alison, Stephen, Sarah, Charlotte and Kathryn who have brought me so much joy.

Author of Chapter 7:
Brian Little, FRCS FRCOphth,
Consultant Ophthalmologist, Department of
Ophthalmology,
Royal Free Hospital, London, UK.

PLEASE READ THE FOLLOWING AGREEMENT CAREFULLY BEFORE USING THIS DVD-ROM PRODUCT. THIS DVD-ROM PRODUCT IS LICENSED UNDER THE TERMS CONTAINED IN THIS DVD-ROM LICENSE AGREEMENT ("Agreement"). BY USING THIS DVD-ROM PRODUCT, YOU, AN INDIVIDUAL OR ENTITY INCLUDING EMPLOYEES, AGENTS AND REPRESENTATIVES ("You" or "Your"), ACKNOWLEDGE THAT YOU HAVE READ THIS AGREEMENT, THAT YOU UNDERSTAND IT, AND THAT YOU AGREE TO BE BOUND BY THE TERMS AND CONDITIONS OF THIS AGREEMENT. ELSEVIER INC. ("Elsevier") EXPRESSLY DOES NOT AGREE TO LICENSE THIS DVD-ROM PRODUCT TO YOU UNLESS YOU ASSENT TO THIS AGREEMENT. IF YOU DO NOT AGREE WITH ANY OF THE FOLLOWING TERMS, YOU MAY, WITHIN THIRTY (30) DAYS AFTER YOUR RECEIPT OF THIS DVD-ROM PRODUCT RETURN THE UNUSED, PIN NUMBER PROTECTED, DVD-ROM PRODUCT, ALL ACCOMPANYING DOCUMENTATION TO ELSEVIER FOR A FULL REFUND.

DEFINITIONS As used in this Agreement, these terms shall have the following meanings:

"Proprietary Material" means the valuable and proprietary information content of this DVD-ROM Product including all indexes and graphic materials and software used to access, index, search and retrieve the information content from this DVD-ROM Product developed or licensed by Elsevier and/or its affiliates, suppliers and licensors.

"DVD-ROM Product" means the copy of the Proprietary Material and any other material delivered on DVD-ROM and any other human-readable or machine-readable materials enclosed with this Agreement, including without limitation documentation relating to the same.

OWNERSHIP This DVD-ROM Product has been supplied by and is proprietary to Elsevier and/or its affiliates, suppliers and licensors. The copyright in the DVD-ROM Product belongs to Elsevier and/or its affiliates, suppliers and licensors and is protected by the national and state copyright, trademark, trade secret and other intellectual property laws of the United States and international treaty provisions, including without limitation the Universal Copyright Convention and the Berne Copyright Convention. You have no ownership rights in this DVD-ROM Product. Except as expressly set forth herein, no part of this DVD-ROM Product, including without limitation the Proprietary Material, may be modified, copied or distributed in hardcopy or machine-readable form without prior written consent from Elsevier. All rights not expressly granted to You herein are expressly reserved. Any other use of this DVD-ROM Product by any person or entity is strictly prohibited and a violation of this Agreement.

SCOPE OF RIGHTS LICENSED (PERMITTED USES) Elsevier is granting to You a limited, non-exclusive, non-transferable license to use this DVD-ROM Product in accordance with the terms of this Agreement. You may use or provide access to this DVD-ROM Product on a single computer or terminal physically located at Your premises and in a secure network or move this DVD-ROM Product to and use it on another single computer or terminal at the same location for personal use only, but under no circumstances may You use or provide access to any part or parts of this DVD-ROM Product on more than one computer or terminal simultaneously.

You shall not (a) copy, download, or otherwise reproduce the DVD-ROM Product in any medium, including, without limitation, online transmissions, local area networks, wide area networks, intranets, extranets and the Internet, or in any way, in whole or in part, except for printing out or downloading nonsubstantial portions of the text and images in the DVD-ROM Product for Your own personal use; (b) alter, modify, or adapt the DVD-ROM Product, including but not limited to decompiling, disassembling, reverse engineering, or creating derivative works, without the prior written approval of Elsevier; (c) sell, license or otherwise distribute to third parties the DVD-ROM Product or any part or parts thereof; or (d) alter, remove, obscure or obstruct the display of any copyright, trademark or other proprietary notice on or in the DVD-ROM Product or on any printout or download of portions of the Proprietary Materials.

RESTRICTIONS ON TRANSFER This License is personal to You, and neither Your rights hereunder nor the tangible embodiments of this DVD-ROM Product, including without limitation the Proprietary Material, may be sold, assigned, transferred or sublicensed to any other person, including without limitation by operation of law, without the prior written consent of Elsevier. Any purported sale, assignment, transfer or sublicense without the prior written consent of Elsevier will be void and will automatically terminate the License granted hereunder.

TERM This Agreement will remain in effect until terminated pursuant to the terms of this Agreement. You may terminate this Agreement at any time by removing from Your system and destroying the DVD-ROM Product. Unauthorized copying of the DVD-ROM Product, including without limitation, the Proprietary Material and documentation, or otherwise failing to comply with the terms and conditions of this Agreement shall result in automatic termination of this license and will make available to Elsevier legal remedies. Upon termination of this Agreement, the license granted herein will terminate and You must immediately destroy the DVD-ROM Product and accompanying documentation. All provisions relating to proprietary rights shall survive termination of this Agreement.

LIMITED WARRANTY AND LIMITATION OF LIABILITY NEITHER ELSEVIER NOR ITS LICENSORS REPRESENT OR WARRANT THAT THE DVD-ROM PRODUCT WILL MEET YOUR REQUIREMENTS OR THAT ITS OPERATION WILL BE UNINTERRUPTED OR ERROR-FREE. WE EXCLUDE AND EXPRESSLY DISCLAIM ALL EXPRESS AND IMPLIED WARRANTIES NOT STATED HEREIN, INCLUDING THE IMPLIED WARRANTIES OF MERCHANTABILITY AND FITNESS FOR A PARTICULAR PURPOSE. IN ADDITION, NEITHER ELSEVIER NOR ITS LICENSORS MAKE ANY REPRESENTATIONS OR WARRANTIES, EITHER EXPRESS OR IMPLIED, REGARDING THE PERFORMANCE OF YOUR NETWORK OR COMPUTER SYSTEM WHEN USED IN CONJUNCTION WITH THE DVD-ROM PRODUCT. WE SHALL NOT BE LIABLE FOR ANY DAMAGE OR LOSS OF ANY KIND ARISING OUT OF OR RESULTING FROM YOUR POSSESSION OR USE OF THE SOFTWARE PRODUCT CAUSED BY ERRORS OR OMISSIONS, DATA LOSS OR CORRUPTION, ERRORS OR OMISSIONS IN THE PROPRIETARY MATERIAL, REGARDLESS OF WHETHER SUCH LIABILITY IS BASED IN TORT, CONTRACT OR OTHERWISE AND INCLUDING, BUT NOT LIMITED TO, ACTUAL, SPECIAL, INDIRECT, INCIDENTAL OR CONSEQUENTIAL DAMAGES. IF THE FOREGOING LIMITATION IS HELD TO BE UNENFORCEABLE, OUR MAXIMUM LIABILITY TO YOU SHALL NOT EXCEED THE AMOUNT OF THE LICENSE FEE PAID BY YOU FOR THE SOFTWARE PRODUCT. THE REMEDIES AVAILABLE TO YOU AGAINST US AND THE LICENSORS OF MATERIALS INCLUDED IN THE SOFTWARE PRODUCT ARE EXCLUSIVE.

If this DVD-ROM Product is defective, Elsevier will replace it at no charge if the defective DVD-ROM Product is returned to Elsevier within sixty (60) days (or the greatest period allowable by applicable law) from the date of shipment.

Elsevier warrants that the software embodied in this DVD-ROM Product will perform in substantial compliance with the documentation supplied in this DVD-ROM Product. If You report a significant defect in performance in writing to Elsevier, and Elsevier is not able to correct same within sixty (60) days after its receipt of Your notification, You may return this DVD-ROM Product, including all copies and documentation, to Elsevier and Elsevier will refund Your money.

YOU UNDERSTAND THAT, EXCEPT FOR THE 60-DAY LIMITED WARRANTY RECITED ABOVE, ELSEVIER, ITS AFFILIATES, LICENSORS, SUPPLIERS AND AGENTS, MAKE NO WARRANTIES, EXPRESSED OR IMPLIED, WITH RESPECT TO THE DVD-ROM PRODUCT, INCLUDING, WITHOUT LIMITATION THE PROPRIETARY MATERIAL, AND SPECIFICALLY DISCLAIM ANY WARRANTY OF MERCHANTABILITY OR FITNESS FOR A PARTICULAR PURPOSE.

If the information provided on this DVD-ROM Product contains medical or health sciences information, it is intended for professional use within the medical field. Information about medical treatment or drug dosages is intended strictly for professional use, and because of rapid advances in the medical sciences, independent verification of diagnosis and drug dosages should be made.

IN NO EVENT WILL ELSEVIER, ITS AFFILIATES, LICENSORS, SUPPLIERS OR AGENTS, BE LIABLE TO YOU FOR ANY DAMAGES, INCLUDING, WITHOUT LIMITATION, ANY LOST PROFITS, LOST SAVINGS OR OTHER INCIDENTAL OR CONSEQUENTIAL DAMAGES, ARISING OUT OF YOUR USE OR INABILITY TO USE THE DVD-ROM PRODUCT REGARDLESS OF WHETHER SUCH DAMAGES ARE FORESEEABLE OR WHETHER SUCH DAMAGES ARE DEEMED TO RESULT FROM THE FAILURE OR INADEQUACY OF ANY EXCLUSIVE OR OTHER REMEDY.

U.S. GOVERNMENT RESTRICTED RIGHTS The DVD-ROM Product and documentation are provided with restricted rights. Use, duplication or disclosure by the U.S. Government is subject to restrictions as set forth in subparagraphs (a) through (d) of the Commercial Computer Restricted Rights clause at FAR 52.22719 or in subparagraph (c)(1)(ii) of the Rights in Technical Data and Computer Software clause at DFARS 252.2277013, or at 252.2117015, as applicable. Contractor/Manufacturer is Elsevier Inc., 360 Park Avenue South, New York, NY 10010 USA.

GOVERNING LAW This Agreement shall be governed by the laws of the State of New York, USA. In any dispute arising out of this Agreement, You and Elsevier each consent to the exclusive personal jurisdiction and venue in the state and federal courts within New York County, New York, USA.

1 Introduction and general issues

Phacoemulsification is the removal of a cataractous lens using ultrasonic energy via a small incision. This technique has developed since the late 1960s and is now the default approach used in most of Europe, Australasia, and the Americas, as well as parts of Asia. The reason it has become so popular is because it provides the facility for rapid rehabilitation with minimal astigmatism in an eye that is left strong following the surgery. It is suitable for day-case surgery and virtually any form of anesthesia (topical, intra-cameral, sub-Tenon's, peribulbar, and general), and it allows for minimal inconvenience for the patient. All this, however, is achievable only with a great deal of expertise and experience. Although the procedure in expert hands can take as little as 5 minutes and an average of probably 15 minutes, the logistic exercise required to get large numbers of patients to the point of having surgery and complete the surgery successfully, with a consistently high standard of good outcomes, is really what this volume is all about. Not only will I examine the surgical techniques themselves, but also the preparation for surgery, the patient pathway, aspects of the theater setup, the instrumentation, and postoperative care and complications. In amongst all this is how to take the cataract out, but all aspects of patient care in the pathway are important. The end product of all this is a pleased patient whose sight is improved, and, although most learning surgeons want to get to the stage of moving the phaco tip inside the eye, the amount of organization, teaching, learning, patience, team effort, and planning that goes into getting to that small part of the process is immense. None of it can be ignored if patient safety and outcomes are to be maximized.

Charles Kelman started clinical trials of phacoemulsification in 1967, after nearly 3 years of research, and began teaching the method to other ophthalmologists in 1969. Even in those days, he was insistent that surgeons knew how to set up the machine before being allowed to use it and had to practice many times on plastic eyes and animal eyes before proceeding to human cases. His course would run for several days and involve didactic lectures as well as practical sessions. Despite early resistance to the technique and somewhat cumbersome equipment, Kelman persevered, as was his nature. Over the course of many years, he not only perfected the technique but influenced a large number of eminent surgeons and spawned an enormous industry, and the technique has helped restore sight to millions of eyes.

Data from randomized controlled trials have helped establish phacoemulsification as a safe technique.[1] This quoted study shows some additional risk with hard cataracts when using phacoemulsification in terms of endothelial cells, but with modern machinery and enhanced software control of the mechanism controlling the phaco needle, shorter phaco times and less endothelial damage are likely. Data collected during the National Cataract Surgery Survey between September and December 1997 showed that 77% of patients in the UK were undergoing phacoemulsification to have their cataract removed.[2] In a study by Riley et al. from New Zealand, carried out between 1997 and 2000, some 97.3% of procedures were by phacoemulsification with foldable lenses.[3]

Teaching and training for phacoemulsification have expanded dramatically since the time of Kelman's original courses, and several different types of model eye are now available as well as a newly developed virtual reality simulator (VR Magic). Phacoemulsification modules have recently been added to training courses.

METHODS

Patient pathway

There are many models described for getting patients through the system, in order to have their cataract removed. All have their advantages and disadvantages, and the relative merits of the different models will be discussed.

LISTING PATIENTS FROM A GENERAL CLINIC

A large number of patients are still processed via a general or more specialized ophthalmic clinic for their cataract surgery. For example, patients attending a glaucoma clinic may need to have their cataract removed both for visual improvement and for monitoring purposes. Quite often, there is not the time in these clinics to carry out the full range of tests necessary for cataract surgery, such as biometry, and patients are therefore often brought back to a preoperative assessment clinic, which means reattending on another day. Figure 1.1 shows a typical patient flow diagram for a patient requiring cataract surgery, coming from a general clinic, and demonstrates that a relatively large number of visits may be required. Similarly, referral from general practice (family medicine) or optometry may follow a similar route (Figure 1.1B). Patients in whom cataract is the primary pathology and who are referred from the primary care sector may follow a more truncated pathway, as shown in Figure 1.2, which is typical of many one-stop cataract clinics.

ONE-STOP CATARACT CLINICS

A number of units in the UK are now taking direct referrals from optometrists via a specially developed form, a copy of

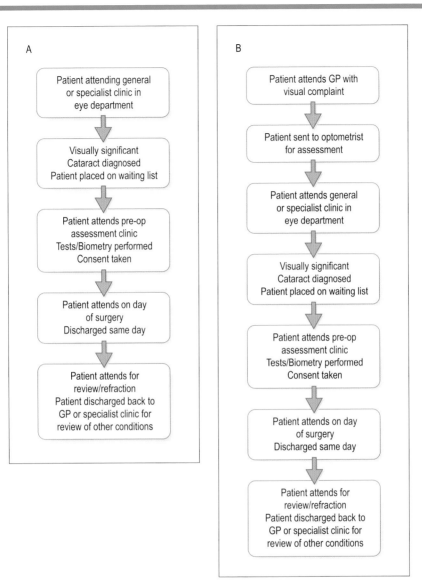

FIGURE 1.1 A typical patient pathway for a patient listed from (**A**) a general ophthalmic clinic and (**B**) via a high-street optometrist or general practitioner (GP) (family doctor).

which is sent to the general practitioner, so that medical details may also be provided about the patient. Patients then attend a hospital, and if the diagnosis is that of cataract alone and they require surgery, they can have all their preoperative investigations and tests at the same clinic visit, be asked for consent, and be given a date for surgery. As can be seen from Figure 1.2, the number of visits is vastly reduced, and it is much more convenient for the patient. Organizationally, this type of clinic requires a large team of people, including preoperative assessment nurses,

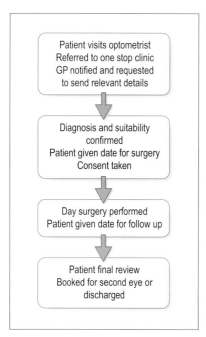

■ **FIGURE 1.2** A truncated pathway, with many fewer visits, for the patient attending through a typical one-stop clinic.

biometry technicians, doctors, and administrative staff, to ensure the smooth passage of patients through the service in a timely fashion.

It is our practice at Stoke Mandeville Hospital, Aylesbury, UK, to talk a patient through the procedure using models and videos; this can be done with a group of patients all at once rather than individually. This will often encourage patients to ask questions, which they might otherwise be afraid to do, and other patients' questions can sometimes address an individual patient's concerns. Showing a video of a typical journey through the unit for a patient having cataract surgery can be very useful and familiarizes the patients with the geography of the unit. In some units, efforts are made to ensure that the preoperative assessment nurse is also available to take the patient to theater and handhold during the procedure, which can be extremely comforting for the patient and give them continuity of care.

SAME-DAY SURGERY

In some UK centers, patients are referred via an optometrist straight to a cataract clinic on the same day. Assuming that patients are suitable and need surgery, they have access to an afternoon operating list on the same day. Although this may be seen as the ultimate in convenience, there are issues about the timing of consent and the need for some patients to think about the decision before surgery, which means that this has not become accepted as routine.

CONSIDERATIONS FOR PEDIATRIC CATARACT SURGERY

The longer-term organization for this sort of surgery is necessarily more involved than for adults, as visual development needs to be taken into account, as well as the physical removal of the cataract. A team of optometrists and orthoptists are involved in the care of the child with developing vision, and it is often extremely hard work for parents, who must be able to comply with the need for aphakic spectacles or contact lenses, and often also the need for occlusion therapy after surgery. However, in terms of the preoperative workup, it is important to have the involvement of pediatrically trained nurses, and showing children around the unit often makes them much more comfortable on the day of surgery, as they are familiar with the surroundings and the staff.

THE CLINIC VISIT

Whichever of the patient pathways above is chosen, the importance of the ophthalmic history and examination cannot be overstressed. Not only is it important to exclude comorbidity, but assessment of the type of cataract is important in terms of anticipating the technique for phacoemulsification later on. Grading the cataract at the slit lamp can give valuable information about the type of surgery required and, in some cases, the type of biometry that might be required. For example, posterior subcapsular cataracts are not easy to assess with the IOL Master, and dense nuclear sclerosis may require recalibrating an ultrasonic biometer to take account of the change in the speed of sound through a harder cataract. A history of trauma or an examination finding of phacodonesis may indicate the need for particular equipment at the time of surgery (iris hooks or capsule tension rings), and comorbidity, such as diabetes, may indicate the need for a different type of lens implant material.

CONSENT

Modern consent forms are necessarily lengthy, and need to be carefully worded so that patients with no medical knowledge can understand the implications of this highly technical, life-changing operation. Clearly, the consent needs to be put into context for individual patients, and it is reasonable to ask them to sign a consent form following a careful explanation of the procedure and its implications on the day of listing them for surgery. It is important that the operation takes place within 3 months of the consent being signed, but signing the consent early has advantages in terms of patients being able to think about the operation and to change their mind, or to ask for further details if required. It also saves time on the day of the operation, and as the theater facilities are such a precious resource, it makes sense to utilize the time on the day of surgery for operating rather than for ward rounds and signing consent forms.

Nurse-led consent is carried out in some areas, and protocols and courses are available for nurses to learn to do this. It is, however, vital that the context of the consent for each patient is taken into account, whoever does the signing, and this may be very different for different groups of patients. For example, the implications for pediatric cataract surgery in terms of continued parental involvement with optical correction, occlusion therapy, attendance at multiple clinics, and long-term follow-up is essential and, while the risks for a one-eyed patient are exactly the same as the risks for a two-eyed patient, the implications of those risks are very different. Risk factors from an individual general health point of view must also be considered; for example, patients on warfarin will need to understand that the risk of hemorrhage at the time of sharp needle anesthesia or expulsive hemorrhage during surgery may be higher. This may, in turn, guide them to a different form of anesthesia, or to reconsider the surgery.

General guidelines for consent form development can be found on the UK Department of Health web site,[4] although local implementation may involve more refined detail and particular complications for particular operations.

BIOMETRY

A detailed account of biometry for intraocular lens implantation will not be given here, as there are several detailed texts on this subject, but suffice to say that accurate biometry is an absolute requirement for successful outcome of cataract surgery, and appropriate equipment and trained staff must be in place for this to occur. The trend nowadays is for non-medical staff to carry out the biometry, but it is imperative that juniors in training learn the technique, and learn its shortcomings and its interpretation, so that appropriate implants can be chosen for individual patients.

It is important that patients bring with them their last set of glasses or a latest refraction, so that an estimation of the optical state of the eye can be made and corroborated with the biometry measurements. It is vital to ensure that appropriate optical correction is obtained and that the optical balance between the eyes is also appropriate. A good way to ensure that this happens is to make it part of the preprinted patient information, which is sent with the outpatient appointment date, requesting the patients to bring this information with them.

Once the biometry has been performed, the selection of a particular implant, make, type, and style, as well as its strength, is critical. In our unit, we use a theater checklist in order to ensure that the appropriate lens and any other surgical implants or devices are available at surgery; Figure 1.3A shows an example of one such form, which, if completed some weeks before surgery, can be used to order

IOL SELECTION ALGORITHM

Operation ....

Pre op glasses prescription   Right ....

                                                Left ....

First eye   Lens power .... Lens type ....

Green card information ....

Any indications for non stock IOL?

Yes   Yes   No

Acrysof lens		High/low power (outside range)

MA60 AC

IOL Master A= 118.9	Ultrasound A= 118.4		Other lens requested (A/C)

Power
(Choose closest to zero on minus side)

Selected IOL

Completed by ....   Date ....

A

Request for special-order intraocular lenses

Date of preop ....   Performed by ....

Patient details	Operation date	Lens type	Lens power

B

■ **FIGURE 1.3** Checklists and forms used to ensure that appropriate intraocular lenses (IOL) are assessed, ordered, and available for surgery. (**A**) IOL selection algorithm. Green card information (e.g. the need for iris hooks or capsule tension rings) is detail taken from the card used for placing a patient on the waiting list. (**B**) Request for special-order intraocular lenses.

non-stock items and ensure that appropriate devices are available on the day of surgery. Ultimately, the surgeon doing the operation needs to select the appropriate implant; quite often, this will need to be done some weeks before surgery so that, if necessary, it can be ordered if it is not a standard stock item. Relying on the selection of implants from a set bank on the day of surgery is inadequate in cases where there is a special requirement.

METHODOLOGIES OF LEARNING

Various approaches to surgical teaching and learning are available, and these are outlined in a paper by Benjamin.[5] Regular and frequent access to the practice of surgical techniques is essential in order for people to progress satisfactorily. This can be done in a wet lab, but access to the operating theater is equally important in order to learn the features and workings of the phacoemulsification machine. It is helpful to scrub with the nurses, and to learn how to set the machine up and how to run it during a procedure under their guidance. This is vital because if there are operational problems during a procedure, it is important to have an approach to being able to solve them, and knowledge of the machine's operational parameters is important. Details of the machine parameters are given in the relevant surgical section.

Special-order lenses (2 weeks' notice required to preorder lens)

Lens	Code	A constant	Range
Alcon Acrysof acrylic PC foldable lens	MA60MA	118.9	−1 to 5 D
Alcon Acrysof acrylic PC foldable lens	MA60AC	118.4 118.9 U/S IOL	6 to 30 D
Vision Matrix Artisan AC claw lens	–	115.0	12 to 25 D
SE Range PC acrylic foldable lens	ACR6D SE	120	31 to 40 D
Trio Len PC acrylic lens	–	115	31 to 35 D

Indications for Acrysof lens

- Age < 50 years
- Diabetes
- Uveitis
- First eye had Acrysof lens
- VR surgery / risk of RD / silicon oil
- High myopia
- Traumatic cataract

Stock lenses

IOL	IOL code	A constant	Size range
Pharmacia silicone foldable IOL	91A	118.3 / 118.7	5.0–30 D with half diopters from 12.5 to 27.5 D
Pharmacia silicone rigid IOL 6.5-mm optic	722C	118.8 / 119.1	8.0–30.0 D with half diopters from 12.5 to 26.5 D
Pharmacia silicone AC IOL	351C	115.2 / 115.5	10.0–27 D with half diopters from 13.5 to 23.5 D
Spectrum acrylic injectable IOL	A2000	118.8 / 119.1	10.0–30.0 D with half diopters from 15.5 to 24.5 D
Pharmacia silicone rigid IOL 5.5-mm optic	812C	117.9	0.0–4.0 D

C

■ **FIGURE 1.3 (C)** Checklist for special-order lenses, indications for Acrysof lenses, and stock lenses. Note that some of the names have changed (Pharmacia is now AMO), and A constants are revised depending on audited outcomes.

REFERENCES

1. Bourne RR, Minassian TC, Dart JK, et al. Effects of cataract surgery on the corneal endothelium: modern phacoemulsification compared with extracapsular cataract surgery. Ophthalmology 2004; 111(4):679–685.
2. Desai P, Minassian TC, Reidy A. National Cataract Surgery Survey 1997–8: report of the results of the clinical outcomes. Br J Ophthalmol 1999; 83(12):1336–1340.
3. Riley AF, Malik TY, Grupcheva CN, et al. Auckland Cataract Study: co-morbidity, surgical techniques and clinical outcomes in a public hospital service. Br J Ophthalmol 2002; 86:105–190.
4. UK Department of Health. Consent key documents. Online. Available: http://www.dh.gov.uk/policyandguidance/healthandsocialcaretopics/consent/consentgeneralinformation
5. Benjamin L. Selection, teaching and training in ophthalmology. Clin Exp Ophthal 2005; 33(5):524–530.

Tools, facilities, and the operating team

THEATER

The operating theater as a facility is one of the most precious resources in any healthcare system in terms of ensuring efficiency and cost-effectiveness.

The operating table and chair

Many modern ophthalmic theaters have trolley beds instead of operating tables; this allows the rapid and smooth interchange of patients between cases, as a patient can be transported from the ward into theater and back to the ward on the same chair. It is important, however, to ensure that any such trolley has adequate facilities for comfortable positioning of the patient and comfortable access for the surgeon, whether operations are done from the 12 o'clock position or from the temporal position. Figure 2.1 shows a typical operating trolley and indicates some of the features that are important for patient comfort. A mechanism for keeping the operating towels off the patient's face is important, and many patients feel more comfortable with air or oxygen delivered under the drapes during the procedure. Easy access to controls for raising and lowering the bed, as well as for tipping and tilting various sections of the table or trolley, is important, and it is vital to ensure that the particular trolley or bed is compatible with the operating microscope in use, so that surgeon comfort is maintained. To establish this, it is important that surgeons sit at a comfortable operating height on their chair, with easy access to the various foot pedals, and, while maintaining a straight back, have the microscope eyepieces positioned so that they are able to operate with their elbows at roughly 90°. While seated in this position, the trolley bed can be brought into position to ensure that it allows the surgeon to maintain his or her comfort, rather than the surgeon having to adjust his or her stool or microscope to accommodate the trolley bed. Clearly, there are conditions under which surgeon comfort may be secondary, for example occasional patients will need to be operated on with the surgeon standing; clearly, this alters the whole positioning ethos.

A number of elderly patients with multiple pathologies will claim not to be able to lie flat. Interestingly, although orthopnea is an important consideration, most patients will tolerate being sat up on the trolley bed and then maneuvered into a relatively flat position for the surgery, while still

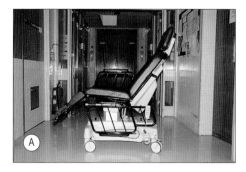
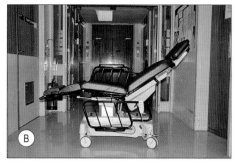
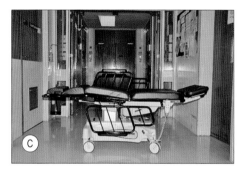
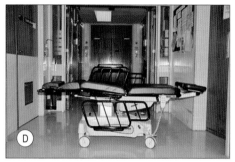
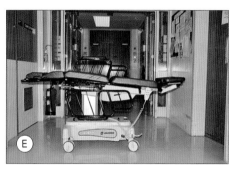
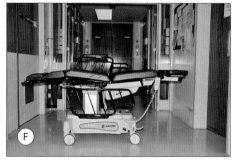

■ **FIGURE 2.1** The different positions a modern trolley chair can adopt. Most patients can be made comfortable on this sort of trolley.

feeling that they are in a seated position. It is therefore important to ensure that the operating table or trolley has this facility. Such a maneuver is shown in Figure 2.2.

Monitoring equipment

Monitoring equipment should be provided for all cases in the form of pulse oximetry. Where sharp needle anesthesia is being used, intravenous access is a sensible precaution. Blood pressure monitoring is also useful, and guidelines for monitoring can be found in the Royal College of Ophthalmologists cataract surgery guideline.[1]

The operating microscope

Modern operating microscopes are optically superb, with very bright light sources but the ability to keep the light

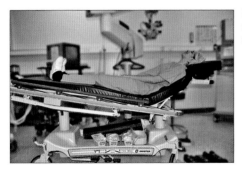

■ **FIGURE 2.2** A patient lying in the seated position can often tolerate 15 or 20 minutes, even if they are orthopneic.

levels low for patient comfort. It is important to set the microscope up to suit the surgeon before the procedure starts, but it should not be forgotten that the assistant also needs to be set up properly and comfortably. It is vital to have a stereoscopic teaching arm on the microscope, so that the assistant can see exactly what is going on. This is especially important if the assistant is trying to perform any surgical maneuvers, apart from wetting the cornea. The ability to alter the assistant's focusing is extremely useful, especially where a presbyopic surgeon is accompanied by a younger trainee, who has much more accommodation. Microscope foot pedals are now programmable, such that the light intensity can be altered, as well as the focus and zoom, and an XY control for the position of the microscope above the patient. All these should be set to zero before the procedure starts, to give maximum range of movement or focus. Microscopes should be equipped with a high-quality, three-chip, CCD camera linked to recording apparatus, and a system for recording each case should be in place, especially where trainees are involved. Various commercial systems are available, and it is important to determine exactly what will be done with the captured images before a purchase is made. If it is envisaged that a lot of video editing will be required for presentations or teaching, then it makes sense to capture in digital video (DV) format, which enables the captured footage to be transferred to a computer for editing. Some capture devices compress the images as they are captured into, for example, MPEG-2 format, and this is much more difficult to get at for editing subsequently. Attention must be paid to the centration and focusing of the microscope during the procedure, as well as the state of the zoom control, in order to get screen-filling detail, which is useful for subsequent viewing or analysis. It is also possible to get interposed stills capture devices, such as that shown in Figure 2.3, and again such images can be used in teaching or presentations. This device has the advantage of a foot-operated pedal for capturing images, which means that the surgeon can capture a picture at any stage of the procedure.

Instruments

There are only a small number of instruments used in any one case for phacoemulsification surgery, but the potential range that can be used is enormous. It is important to know the names and designs of the instruments used and to be able to ask for them by name during a case, especially if things are not going according to plan. Again, scrubbing with the nurses enables junior ophthalmologists to learn the order of the operation and the names of the instruments very quickly, and also gives them instruction in how to handle and manipulate the instruments. Instruments must also be passed to the operating surgeon the right way round at the right time, and this helps the learning curve. A typical cataract set is seen in Figure 2.4. It is said that a good scrub nurse will give you the instrument you need, not necessarily the one you ask for. Certainly, very experienced scrub nurses can anticipate events well in advance of them happening and have the appropriate instrumentation ready. It is sometimes helpful for learning surgeons to be made to ask for an instrument by name in order to encourage them to learn what the instrument is, rather than being given something that they are unfamiliar with and that they may not know how to use.

Learning about instruments is another useful task that can be accomplished in a skills center, as well as how to use them and what they are called.

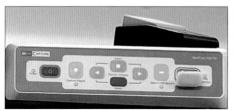

■ **FIGURE 2.3** A stills image capture device with foot pedal, which operates the frame grabber to select stills from the operating camera at any stage during the operation.

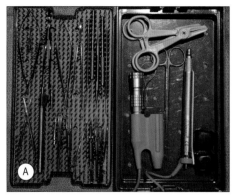

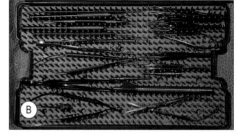

■ **FIGURE 2.4** (**A**) A typical cataract set, showing the phaco handpiece and associated instrumentation. (**B**) A close-up of the microsurgical instruments. The names of these should be learned by trainee surgeons.

Theater team

A scrub nurse and a runner are essential to the efficient running of an operating list. Also useful for local anesthesia is a person to hold the hand of the patient, through whom communication from the patient to the surgeon can be made. In the centers where nurses see the patients in the outpatient department, bring them into theater, and hold their hand during the case, there are strong anecdotal reports that the patients feel in better communication throughout the operation and less isolated. It is also very useful, if things are not going according to plan, to have a person holding the patient's hand who can, with appropriate communication, take the patient's attention away from the technicalities of the procedure. It is very useful before a complicated case to meet with the scrub nurse and the runner to go through a list of instruments that might potentially be used during the case. It is sensible to have equipment such as iris hooks or capsule tension rings available on the side in the operating theater in case they are needed, rather than having to go and look for them in an urgent situation. Similarly, access to and knowledge of the anterior vitrectomy equipment should be second nature. If required, such equipment should be asked for in a steady tone of voice so as not to alarm the patient. Efficient patient flow through the theater is entirely dependent on a good team spirit, and acknowledgment of the importance of different members of the team is essential.

Recording equipment

Recorded operations provide an extremely valuable learning and teaching tool. A counsel of perfection is to record every case; while this may not be possible for all surgery, it is certainly possible to record an entire list of cataract operations. In order to obtain high-quality recordings, it is essential to have a high-quality camera. Although there are a number of good single-chip cameras on the market, it is a distinct advantage in quality terms to have a three-chip camera to make the recordings. These can easily be attached to a number of different types of recording device. Exactly which type of device is used depends a little on what the records are used for. If they are simply going to be reviewed, then virtually any medium is acceptable. However, if further use is to be made of the recordings, for example editing them for teaching purposes, then it is an advantage to capture the material on to mini DV tape, as subsequent editing on a computer is very much easier to organize. If images are captured on to VHS videotape, the quality tends to be lower. If primary capture is on to mechanisms containing DVD drives, then the source material tends to be compressed, which makes subsequent editing much more difficult. Figure 2.5 shows a recording stack in an operating theater, which has the facility for VHS, mini DV, and digital stills recording, all of which can be used for subsequent review or edited for teaching purposes.

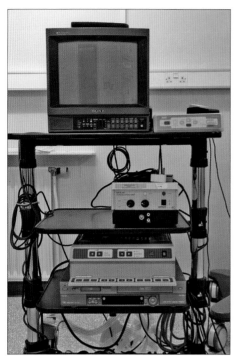

■ **FIGURE 2.5** A recording stack that has the availability of VHS and mini digital videotape recording, as well as stills capture, the interface for white balance and color balance, and exposure controls.

By routinely recording cataract cases, it is possible to build up an excellent collection of teaching material, both in terms of straightforward surgery and complication management.

PHACOEMULSIFICATION MACHINE

The purpose of these machines is to provide surgeons with a configurable, controllable surgical tool, which suits their particular mode of operating. Modern machines are highly programmable and configurable, and it is essential that surgeons are familiar with their machine before attempting phacoemulsification. This is best learned in the wet lab, where a range of options can be tried, and familiarity with the various modalities and warning sounds can be gained. It is particularly important to learn what an individual surgeon's settings are programmed to do, as it may be that, for example, the foot pedal is configured in a particular way such that whereas one would expect reflux from the tip of the phaco probe, it actually causes the machine to go into another programmed mode. Clearly, this can be very dangerous if the exact parameters are not known. Therefore, although a number of surgeons who teach usually suggest that their trainees use the same settings as they do, it is imperative that the trainee also knows of any particular programmed differences.

A brief guide to the different types of machines available and the different control options that are possible will be

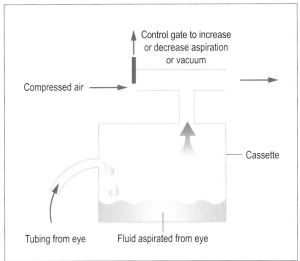

■ **FIGURE 2.6** A Venturi pump. Compressed air is blown across tubing, via a variable gate, producing a Venturi effect and vacuum in the cassette, which draws fluid from the eye into the cassette. The foot pedal controls the opening of the variable gate to vary the vacuum and aspiration.

given here, but there is no substitute for learning the particular machine that one is using in the wet lab. Most companies will provide this sort of training to units that purchase their apparatus; indeed, it should be a requirement of the purchasing order that this is available.

Pump types

Figures 2.6, 2.7, and 2.8 show the three main pump types: Venturi, peristaltic, and diaphragmatic. Largely, nowadays, the first two are the most popular in production, and the principles of their operation will be given.

Principles of fluid flow through the eye

The purpose of the pump in the phaco machine is to facilitate flow of fluid through the eye. The concepts of inflow and outflow must be appreciated in order to understand how the machine is helping to control the fluid dynamics. Figure 2.9 shows a typical setup, with a phaco probe in the eye and the various parts of the circuit labeled to show fluid dynamics during a procedure. Before the details of the various pump types are given, an explanation of the foot pedal is in order to explain how the machine is controlled.

Foot pedal

A typical foot pedal is shown in Figure 2.10. Figure 2.11 shows the three main positions of the foot pedal. These are common to all phaco machines, although some have variations on this theme. For example, the dual linear control of the Storz Millennium machine allows sideways movement of the pedal in position 3, and this can be programmed to do different things. Essentially, position 1 opens a pinch valve on the phaco machine, allowing fluid from the infusion bottle into the tubing, which is attached to the phaco probe

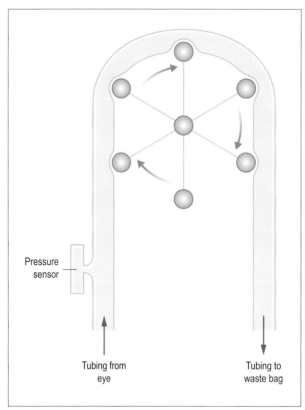

■ **FIGURE 2.7** A peristaltic pump. As the pump turns, the rollers milk fluid through the tubing and aspirate it from the eye and into the waste bag. Modern machines have pressure-sensing devices on the tubing to help control flow and alleviate problems such as post-occlusion surge.

Pressure sensor

Tubing from eye

Tubing to waste bag

in the eye. The flow of this fluid is gravity-fed and, with the phaco probe out of the eye, a steady flow of fluid will come out of irrigating ports on the side of the infusion sleeve. For beginning surgeons, it is useful to ask the nursing staff to switch on free flow of fluid, so that position 1 becomes inoperable and fluid is flowing all the time. This means that, if the operating surgeon's foot inadvertently comes out of position 1, fluid will still be able to flow into the eye, and the anterior chamber will not collapse. Position 2 switches on the pump and, in the case of a peristaltic pump, starts it turning at a preset speed to aspirate or draw fluid out of the eye at a predetermined rate. For example, 25 mL/min can be set and, as position 2 is reached, the pump starts turning and fluid is drawn out of the eye, or aspirated, from the anterior chamber by the pump and replaced by the gravity-fed fluid from the bottle. This is a steady state, and inflow should equal outflow at this point. If the infusion bottle is too low, then it is possible that, with a very high aspiration rate set, the anterior chamber will collapse. It is therefore important to make sure that the inflow, which is fluid replacing that being aspirated out of the eye, is adequate. Position 3 of the foot pedal provides electric current to the handpiece, and causes the piezo electric crystals of the handpiece to vibrate at a set frequency depending on the

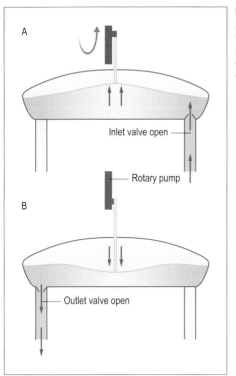

■ FIGURE 2.8 A diaphragm pump. A small rotary pump drives the diaphragm up and down. (**A**) On the upstroke, fluid is sucked in through an inlet valve. (**B**) The inlet valve closes on the downstroke, while the outlet valve opens, allowing fluid out through the other side of the mechanism. These pumps have rather fallen out of favor now.

A

Inlet valve open

Rotary pump

B

Outlet valve open

particular machine (between 28 000 and 40 000 Hz); these are linked to the phaco needle, which vibrates at that frequency. Phaco power is the distance that the needle travels with each vibration; 100% power would be the maximum excursion that the needle can travel with each vibration. Fifty percent phaco power would mean that the needle is traveling half its maximum possible distance with each vibration.

The various sidepieces on the foot pedal can be programmed for different functions. Usually, one is set to cause reflux so that, if tissue is drawn into the phaco needle, pressing the reflux button can blow fluid back into the eye; this is often accomplished by temporarily reversing the pump. Other side panels can be used to cycle through the programme modes on the phaco machine. It is advisable to operate without operating shoes or boots, as greater sensitivity of foot pedal control will be obtained.

Pump types

An excellent account of phacodynamics can be found in Barry Seibel's book.[2]

Peristaltic pump

Also known as flow pumps, these devices depend on mechanical movement of rollers against silicone tubing, which

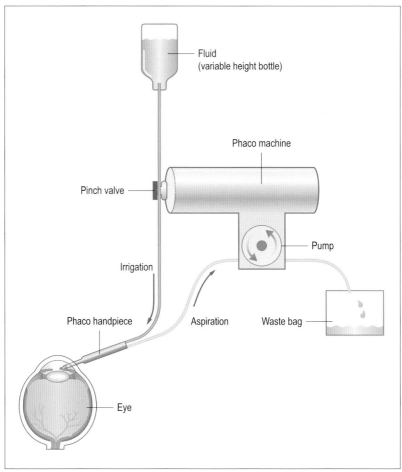

Fluid
(variable height bottle)

Phaco machine

Pinch valve

Pump

Irrigation

Phaco handpiece

Aspiration

Waste bag

Eye

■ **FIGURE 2.9** A typical setup of the phaco probe in the eye. The fluid dynamics diagram shows that, as the pump in the phaco machine aspirates fluid from the eye into the waste bag, it is replaced by a fluid flowing in from the irrigation bottle.

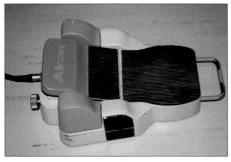

■ **FIGURE 2.10** A foot pedal from an Alcon Legacy machine. The side panels are programmable for functions such as backflow and for cycling through the preset memories.

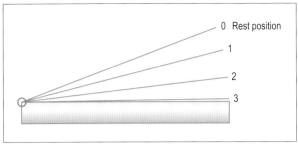

■ **FIGURE 2.11** The typical positions of a phaco foot pedal. Position 1 opens the pinch valve, allowing irrigation. Position 2 switches on the pump in the phaco machine, causing fluid to be aspirated from the eye. Position 3 supplies current to the phaco handpiece to drive the phaco needle.

squeezes fluid along the tube. This is likened to peristaltic movement of the gut.

Regardless of the pump type, manufacturers have moved more recently to providing systems that give much higher vacuums in order that nuclear fragments can be removed with much less phaco power being used. This so-called phaco-assisted aspiration depends on having high vacuums and a relatively rapid rise time, which can be accomplished on most machines now. The rise time is the time taken for the preset vacuum on the machine to reach its maximum preset value. In the peristaltic machine, vacuum is obtained only once the tip of the phaco needle is occluded, as when this happens the pump continues to turn and a negative pressure is developed in the tubing, causing a rise in vacuum. Modern machines have very non-compliant tubing of a relatively small diameter, which allows a rapid rise in vacuum without collapsing the tubing wall. The maximum preset vacuum can be varied between 50 and 400 mmHg. Table 2.1 shows a number of different settings that can be used for different nuclear removal techniques. In a peristaltic system, as the rollers of the peristaltic pump turn, once the phaco tip is occluded and vacuum rises, the preset maximum vacuum is maintained by a venting system, preventing any further rise. By increasing the aspiration rate, the flow of fluid through the anterior chamber is increased; this produces an effect called 'followability', which describes the ease with which fragments move in the flow or current of fluid around the anterior chamber and reach the phaco needle. This flow pattern is shown in Figure 2.12. Modern machines using low compliance tubing and high vacuum settings can be prone to post-occlusion surge, a situation that arises as a nuclear fragment that has blocked the phaco tip is removed, and in which there is a sudden increase in the flow of fluid up the phaco needle. There are a number of mechanical and electronic devices built into modern machines to reduce this phenomenon.

Venturi systems
Venturi pumps differ from peristaltic pumps by virtue of the fact that some negative pressure is present in the system at all times. The aspiration rate and vacuum are combined into

TABLE 2.1 Suggested settings for different nuclear removal techniques

Technique	Parameter	Divide and conquer	Phaco chop, stop and chop	Chip and flip	Vertical chop
Sculpting	Vacuum (mmHg)	30–60	30–60	30–60	No sculpting phase
	Aspiration rate (mL/min)	25–30	25–30	20–25	
	Phaco power (%)	50	50	50	
Fragment removal	Vacuum (mmHg)	350	350	350	350
	Aspiration rate (mL/min)	25–35	25–35	25–35	25–35
	Phaco power (%)	50 (pulsed, 10 Hz)	50 (pulsed, 10 Hz)	50 (pulsed, 10 Hz)	50

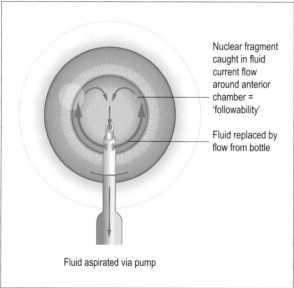

Nuclear fragment caught in fluid current flow around anterior chamber = 'followability'

Fluid replaced by flow from bottle

Fluid aspirated via pump

■ **FIGURE 2.12** Diagram showing 'followability', or the ease with which a fragment is brought to the phaco tip. Think of the current as pushing the fragment toward the tip, and the aspiration or vacuum as pulling it.

one setting and entirely dependent on the flow of air across the opening in the Venturi pump. This is what is controlled by depressing the foot pedal further in position 2. These pumps are therefore also known as vacuum pumps. It is said that followability with these pumps is better. They certainly have a more rapid vacuum rise time, which, in skilled hands, can speed up the process of fragment removal, but of course the corollary of this is that, in inexperienced hands, there is a danger that things happen extremely quickly and the whole environment in the anterior chamber is less controllable.

In order to develop the very high rates of flow across the Venturi pump required to operate it, a compressor or compressed air cylinder supply is needed to run these machines.

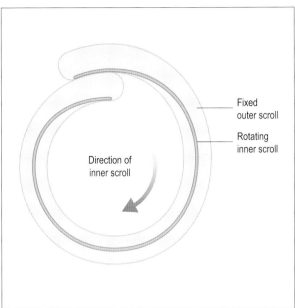

■ **FIGURE 2.13** A scroll pump. This type of pump can mimic a peristaltic or Venturi system. It allows flow control *or* vacuum control depending on the variability of pump rotation speed. Rotation at a constant preset speed produces peristaltic-like behavior and, by varying the speed, variable vacuum is obtained.

Fixed outer scroll

Rotating inner scroll

Direction of inner scroll

Diaphragmatic pump
The movement of fluid through these pumps is generated by the up and down motion of a deformable diaphragm. The fluid dynamic characteristics of these pumps are somewhere between those of the Venturi and peristaltic systems.

Scroll pump
Found in some modern machines, this is a pump that can be made to mimic both peristaltic and Venturi systems. Figure 2.13 shows the construction of a scroll pump, which utilizes an inner scroll rotating against a fixed outer one. To mimic a flow, or peristaltic pump, the rotation of the inner scroll is kept at a constant preset speed, but, by varying the speed, a variable vacuum can be obtained. This is similar to the Venturi pump.

Fluid dynamics
The purpose of the aforementioned pump technologies is to produce controllable flow in a stable anterior chamber during cataract removal. During any sculpting technique, details of which are discussed in subsequent chapters, the main useful parameter is flow of fluid in via the infusion sleeve and out via the hollow phaco needle. It is this current flow that removes the nuclear fragments as they are sculpted, and in a peristaltic system it is the aspiration rate that controls the flow. In a Venturi system, vacuum and aspiration are combined as one parameter, producing the same effect. When nuclear fragments are removed, the vacuum is utilized to hold on to pieces of cataract as they are phacoemulsified. During this part of the procedure, faster flow and higher

vacuum settings are used to attract and hold on to nuclear fragments as the tip of the phaco needle breaks them up. The movement of the phaco needle generates heat, which is why cooling infusion fluid is required and any interruption to the flow of fluid can produce a phaco burn by allowing significant heat rise from the vibrating needle. For this reason, modern machines have a variety of ways in which to modify the needle vibrations, including pulsed and burst mode.

Phaco tip technology

Nuclear fragmentation is produced by two main effects.

1. A jack hammer effect. This is similar to the effect seen with a jack hammer used for breaking up tarmac on road surfaces. The very rapid to and fro movement of the needle tip mechanically breaks up the cataractous lens.
2. Cavitation. This effect can be seen just ahead of the advancing tip of the vibrating needle as a clear zone. It is thought to be produced by the production of micro-bubbles, which by expanding and collapsing very rapidly develop very high pressures and temperatures just ahead of the vibrating needle.

Both these effects will be influenced by the shape, size, and cross-sectional area of the vibrating needle; this has led to the development of different needle types.

Needle types

The standard phacoemulsification needle has a 30° angled tip, but 15 and 45° angles are also available. The 15° angled tip will be easier to occlude but presents a smaller total cutting surface area to the cataract and may be slower with harder cataracts. The 45° tip cuts more effectively because of the larger surface area of the needle tip, but it is more difficult to occlude. A good compromise is a 30° tip. Angled tips such as the Kelman needle are also available. These tips present a relatively large surface area to the cataract for increased cutting and cavitation, but the bend is also supposed to produce internal cavitation to prevent occlusion internally. Other needles have been produced with smaller openings and a greater mass to produce more cavitation, but there is a danger of occlusion with these smaller-diameter needles. Figure 2.14 shows some of the needles available.

Phaco modes

Straightforward phacoemulsification produces needle vibrations at a preset frequency and a preset maximum power. Position 3 on the foot pedal can be set to linear, in which case increasing depression of the foot pedal produces increasing phaco power up to the preset limit; this is known as surgeon control. It can also be set to panel control, in which, as soon as position 3 is reached, full preset phaco power is delivered to the needle tip. The needle vibrations produce quite an intense heat rise, which experimentally can be shown to be as much as 37° in 2 min without cooling

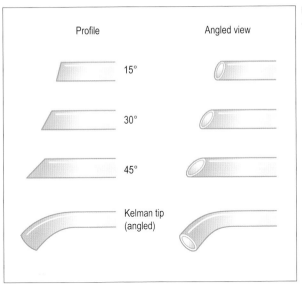

■ **FIGURE 2.14** Some of the different phaco tips available.

fluid. This is the cause of phaco burns; when the tip is occluded, fluid flow is temporarily stopped and the needle continues to vibrate, generating heat. For this reason, a number of technologies have been developed to modify the needle vibrations and reduce the heat and energy generated.

Pulsed mode

In pulsed mode, the needle vibrations are switched off intermittently at a preset frequency. For example, 10 Hz means that the needle will deliver phaco power for a set amount of time: 10 times a second. This pulsing of energy delivery can be heard as an intermittent buzzing. The advantages of this are that heat dissipation and cooling can occur in between the sets of vibrations, and there is also less tendency for the phaco needle to push fragments away, which can occur during straightforward phacoemulsification.

Burst mode

In burst mode, the frequency of the pulses is altered as the foot pedal is further depressed in position 3. Eventually, as the foot pedal reaches the bottom of its travel, full phaco, with no interruptions, is achieved.

White Star technology

This method of phaco delivery is found in the Allergan White Star machine. This technology can be thought of as a type of pulsed mode, but with each individual pulse broken up into much higher frequency pulsed vibrations. Figure 2.15 shows the difference between pulsed mode and White Star mode. Each duty cycle of 500 ms within each second is further broken up into episodes of 10-ms pulse with a 10-ms rest, five times every 100 ms. This puts much less energy

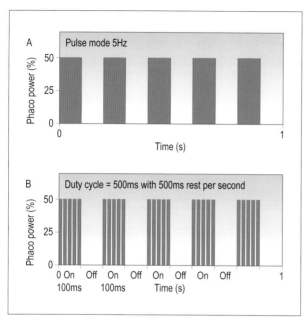

FIGURE 2.15 The difference between (**A**) ordinary pulsed mode (5 Hz) and (**B**) White Star technology (duty cycle 500 ms with 500-ms rest per second).

into the eye and allows phacoemulsification to proceed with no cooling sleeve.

Neosonix

With this device, produced by Alcon, a sideways rotational movement of 2° occurs at 100 Hz, as well as the usual longitudinal oscillation of the phaco tip. This provides greater mechanical advantage when breaking up hard cataracts, but has to utilize a handpiece with a larger diameter, as it houses a small electric motor.

SUMMARY

Modern machines are designed to provide a safe, stable environment in which to remove a cataract. Learning the parameters of the specific machine and pump type, as well as being able to control the fluid flow and tip dynamics, are essential components of safe phacoemulsification surgery.

REFERENCES

1. Royal College of Ophthalmologists. Cataract surgery guidelines 2005. Online. Available: http://www.rcophth.ac.uk

2. Seibel BS. Phacodynamics: mastering the tools and techniques of phacoemulsification. 3rd edn. Thorofare: Slack; 1999.

3 Anesthesia for cataract surgery

Most cataract surgery is carried out under local anesthesia and as a day case. The original driver for this was the perceived cost of an inpatient stay versus that of a day case procedure. The costs are actually fairly similar, and the exact combination of inpatient or day case, and local or general anesthesia, should be tailored to suit the individual patient. Clearly, a 90-year-old living on her or his own with severe respiratory problems and Parkinson disease would present a completely different set of challenges to those of a 6-month-old baby with congenital cataract. It is important, therefore, to have access to the full range of anesthetic facilities in order to provide a complete service. A good account of the relative safety of different types of anesthesia is given in *Cataract Surgery* by Coombes and Gartry.[1]

It is not only important to consider the safety of the patient, but also the comfort of the surgeon in coming to a mutual decision about what type of anesthesia to use. It is often easier to control the conditions inside the eye with a general anesthetic with known levels of P_{CO_2} and the ability to hyperventilate in order to soften the globe. Thus, for a one-eyed patient with a traumatic partly subluxed cataract, general anesthesia may present several advantages. On the other hand, the convenience of local anesthesia and lack of systemic upset are the oft-quoted advantages of a local anesthetic.

LOCAL ANESTHESIA

Retrobulbar block

Once the standard form of local anesthesia, retrobulbar block has now been replaced by much safer methods. The long retrobulbar needle was associated with a number of potentially serious complications, including retrobulbar hemorrhage, optic nerve injury, and intrameningeal injection of anesthetic, which could lead to brainstem anesthesia and death. Globe perforations were also reported.

The technique of retrobulbar injection involves asking patients to stare at a point directly above them (assuming they are lying down). There was a vogue for asking the patient to look upward as the injection was given, but elegant studies using computed tomography demonstrated that this actually causes the optic nerve to be positioned in the way of the needle.[2] Having advanced the needle through the anterior third of the orbit, sometimes a small resistance could be felt as the needle traversed the orbital septum. At this point, the needle was angled more acutely upward into the muscle cone and the anesthetic delivered.

The effectiveness of retrobulbar as compared with peribulbar block is probably no different. However, as the risks of retrobulbar block are higher, in this author's view the technique should be avoided in favor of peribulbar block or sub-Tenon's anesthesia.

Topical

It is said that if a patient is suitable for local anesthesia, then he or she is probably suitable for topical anesthesia. Some studies report some discomfort for patients during surgery with topical anesthesia alone, but others, such as that by O'Brien et al.,[3] suggest that even patients undergoing pupil-stretching maneuvers did not experience significant discomfort. Topical anesthetic agents can be used alone or in combination with intracameral, preservative-free lidocaine (lignocaine). Different authors suggest the use of either 0.5 or 1% intracameral lidocaine, but there are as yet no long-term studies on the potential endothelial toxicity of this substance. Undoubtedly, intracameral lidocaine provides better analgesia, especially if manipulation of the iris or changes in pressure in the anterior chamber occur. Proxymetacaine, benoxinate, or amethocaine can be used, although the last of these can occasionally cause epithelial clouding. Movement of the globe is unaffected by these agents; this can sometimes be useful in asking the patient to look in a particular direction, but can also be counter-productive if the patient moves during a critical part of the procedure. The intensity of the microscope light should be kept as low as possible to avoid photophobia when initially placing the microscope over the eye if topical agents alone are used.

Peribulbar block

Injections of 2% plain lidocaine or bupivacaine 0.5% can be used for peribulbar anesthesia using a 25-mm, 25-gauge needle (Fig. 3.1). The eye is kept in the primary position during passage of the needle. It is important to withdraw the plunger of the syringe after passage of the needle to ensure that the vascular compartment has not been entered. It is also reasonable to ask a patient to gently move the eye to the right and left to make sure that the globe has not been snagged before injecting the local anesthetic. There is some evidence that bupivacaine causes extraocular muscle toxicity; for this reason, some surgeons use lidocaine 2% on its own. There is conflicting evidence about the use of hyaluronidase, which is supposed to ensure a greater spread of the anesthetic, and many surgeons have abandoned its use. However, although it probably does not give any advantage in terms of anesthesia, it does appear to have some protective effect in terms of diplopia.[4] Between 2

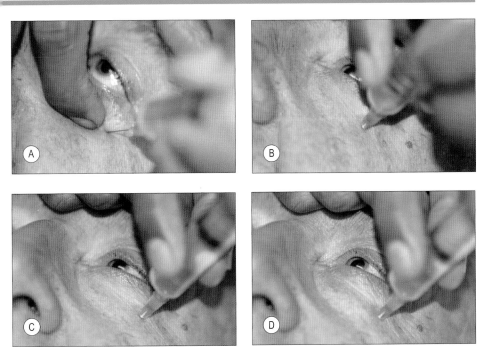

■ **FIGURE 3.1.** (**A**) The orbital margin is palpated, and the orange needle directed toward the periosteum. As it meets the periosteum, it is angled more vertically into the orbit. (**B**) Once the needle has reached its correct depth, the patient is asked to gently move his or her eyes side to side to ensure that the globe is not tethered. (**C**) The plunger on the syringe is withdrawn to ensure that the needle is not within a vascular compartment. (**D**) Between 2 and 5 mL of anesthetic is injected into the anterior orbit.

and 5 mL of local anesthetic agent is injected into the anterior orbit. Larger volumes should be avoided, as they can produce significant pressure behind the globe, which can cause complications during surgery.

The use of a Honan's balloon is advocated by some. This is placed on the eye for a few minutes after the administration of anesthetic to compress the globe and effectively soften it, but it is possible to exert high pressures with this device if it is not properly positioned. Techniques that make the injection of anesthetic comfortable are first, to warm the solution to body temperature; second, to use isotonic solution (isotonic lidocaine is now available); and third, to inject it slowly.

Sub-Tenon's anesthesia

This technique has gained popularity recently because, although it does not provide such good akinesia as a peribulbar does, it provides excellent anesthesia and is very much safer from the point of view of avoiding sharp needles. As little as 1 mL of anesthetic can be given. Because of its close proximity to the ciliary ganglion, it can induce excellent anesthesia very rapidly. Larger volumes will induce akinesia if 10–15 min is allowed to elapse. The technique is an excellent one to use in patients who are anticoagulated or highly myopic, for whom sharp needle anesthesia may be more of a risk. Figure 3.2 shows administration of sub-Tenon's anesthetic in the inferonasal quadrant; this is performed via a small nick in the conjunctivum and Tenon's with blunt dissection onto the sclera before insertion of the blunt cannula. Initial resistance may be felt as the injection is given, but if the cannula is retracted 1 mm and then injection commenced while the cannula is being re-advanced the spread of local anesthetic will be relatively easy.

A Honan's balloon can be used as for a peribulbar injection (Fig. 3.3).

Between 1 and 2 mL of anesthesia (lidocaine 2%) is usually sufficient for excellent anesthesia. If akinesia is also required, a larger volume should be administered (up to 4–5 mL) and it is necessary to wait 10–15 min before akinesia is obtained. As regards the advantages with particular anesthetic agents, a study by Koh and Cammack showed no difference in clinical effect between the two solutions.[5]

Intracameral anesthesia

Intracameral local anesthetic has been added to viscoelastic ophthalmic surgical devices (VisThesia) and is also used in the balanced salt infusion fluid to essentially provide anesthesia of the iris during surgery. A paper by Poyales-Galan and Pirazzoli suggests that VisThesia, which is a mixture of sodium hyaluronate 0.3% and lidocaine hydrochloride 2%, does not induce additional toxicity or result in increased endothelial cell loss when compared with other similar anesthesia-free ophthalmic viscosurgical devices.[6] However, long-term studies on the use of infused lidocaine 2% are not currently available, and it is clearly important to establish the safety of such drugs intracamerally even though their effectiveness is proven.

Monitoring

Monitoring of the electrocardiogram, pulse oximetry, and establishing intravenous access are all important for sharp needle anesthesia. It is also usually standard to have monitoring of the blood pressure during the procedure. This can be distressing for some patients, although a careful explanation of what is happening often allays their fears.

Sedation

Intravenous midazolam 1–2 mg is often adequate to sedate anxious patients. It is also a useful technique for patients with dementia who are not completely cooperative but in whom a general anesthetic would be more of a risk.

There are risks if the sedation is incomplete, in that the patient will suddenly become aroused halfway through the procedure, and it does require an experienced anesthetist to get the level of sedation right. Over-sedation can also be a

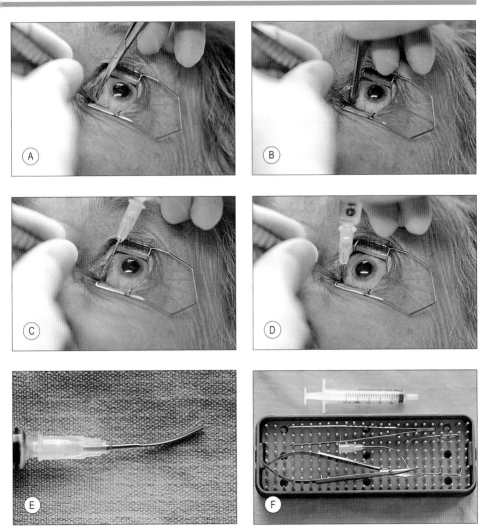

■ **FIGURE 3.2.** (**A**) A small nick is made in the inferomedial quadrant, with the patient looking upward and outward, using a Westcott scissors and Moorfields forceps. The incision is made through both conjunctiva and Tenon's. (**B**) Blunt section, using a spreading action with the Westcott scissors beneath the Tenon's layer, locates the surface of the sclera. (**C**) A disposable sub-Tenon's cannula is used to enter the sub-Tenon's space. (**D**) The curved shape of the cannula allows relatively deep passage around the globe, and injection can be started. Initial resistance may be felt, after which the cannula can be withdrawn 1 mm, injection restarted, and then the cannula advanced further. (**E**) A gently curved, flattened, sub-Tenon's cannula. (**F**) A preprepared sterilized sub-Tenon's kit comprising a lid speculum, a pair of Westcott spring scissors, and Moorfields forceps, to which has been added a disposable sub-Tenon's cannula.

problem in terms of airway obstruction; careful monitoring and anesthetic input is imperative.

GENERAL ANESTHESIA

Recent advances in short-acting drug availability and airway maintenance with laryngeal mask airways have made general anesthetic day case surgery a realistic possibility for

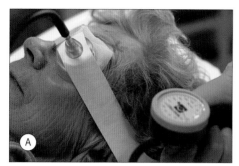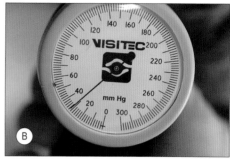

■ **FIGURE 3.3. (A)** Honan's balloon in position. The one shown is a disposable version, held in place with an adjustable paper strip. **(B)** The pressure in a Honan's balloon is maintained at around 30 mmHg for 10 min.

most patients. Such agents include atracurium and vecuronium, which are muscle relaxants with a short half-life; alfentanil, which is a short-acting opioid analgesic; and propofol, which is a short-acting induction agent that can also be used for maintenance anesthesia. All ensure that patients are awake and alert enough to go home on the day of surgery. Similarly, inhalation anesthesia, such as with sevoflurane, is not only rapid in its onset of action but also wears off quickly, again allowing early discharge of patients following general anesthesia. The main advantages of general anesthesia, from the patient's point of view, are complete anesthesia and no memory of the surgery itself, and its use takes away the obvious difficulties that local anesthesia would cause for patients who cannot communicate or are uncooperative. From the surgeon's perspective, it allows a greater control of the intraocular pressure, as, by hyperventilating the patient, choroidal blood flow can be reduced and intraocular pressure lowered. It also allows for freedom of speech during training, which may mean a more relaxed training episode, and ensures a completely immobile eye and patient.

The potential complications are numerous but rare. With short-acting agents, as outlined above, day case general anesthesia is a method of choice in a number of patients.

REFERENCES

1. Coombes A, Gartry D. Fundamentals of clinical ophthalmology: cataract surgery. London: BMJ Books; 2003.
2. Unsold R, Stanley J, DeGroot J. The CT topography of retrobulbar anaesthesia. Anatomic–clinical correlation of complications and suggestion of a modified technique. Graefes Arch Clin Ophthalmol 1981; 217:125–136.
3. O'Brien PD, Fitzpatrick P, Power W. Patient pain during stretching of small pupils in phacoemulsification performed using topical anesthesia. J Cataract Refract Surg 2005; 31(9):1760–1763.
4. Hamada S, Devys JM, Xuan TH, et al. Role of hyaluronidase in diplopia after peribulbar anaesthesia for cataract surgery. Ophthalmology 2005; 112(5):879–882.
5. Koh JW, Cammack R. Sub-Tenon's block in cataract surgery—a comparison of 1% ropivacaine and a mixture of 2% lignocaine and 0.5% bupivacaine. Anaesth Intensive Care 2005; 33(5):597–600.
6. Poyales-Galan F, Pirazzoli G. Clinical evaluation of endothelial cell decrease with VisThesia in phacoemulsification surgery. J Cataract Refract Surg 2005; 31(11):2157–2161.

4 Preparation for surgery

The patient should arrive at the surgical unit in plenty of time to be properly prepared for surgery. The preoperative checklist should include agreeing the patient's details, the type of operation and its laterality, and that the consent form has been signed. The type of anesthesia that is to be administered should be checked, as well as details of fasting if necessary. An approximate time on the list should be established, so that the patient can visit the toilet preoperatively; a full bladder on the operating table is a common cause of patient and surgeon discomfort! Dilating drops should be instilled into the appropriate eye. If it is established practice on the unit concerned to mark the eye for operation, this should be done with a suitable marking pen.

PREOPERATIVE EVALUATION

History taking preoperatively is vital to ascertain the nature and extent of visual loss and what functional visual limitations are being experienced by the patient. Only then can a realistic expectation be given to the patient about the possible outcomes, and it should be emphasized which symptoms can and cannot be ascribed to the cataract itself. Quality of vision is very important to the patient, and numerous studies have described the inadequacy of Snellen acuity as a measure of outcome success. Patient-assessed outcomes have been validated and assessed and should perhaps be in more widespread use, particularly for research into new styles of implant.[1,2] Younger patients in particular may need specific counseling about dysphotopsia and night vision problems such as glare and haloes (see Ch. 16, *Wavefront aberrometry and cataract surgery*).

The cause of the cataract is often ascertained during history taking, for example it is useful to elucidate a history of trauma, as anticipating loose zonules or vitreous presenting around the edge of the loose lens at surgery can be extremely useful. The history will also guide the physical examination with respect to the need for gonioscopy to look for angle recession after trauma; testing the crystalline lens for phacodonesis, which indicates loose or lax zonules, and a dense cataract after trauma, or indeed in any case, would necessitate a B-scan ultrasound to check the status of the retina.

An estimation of the pupil size after dilation in the clinic can give guidance as to potential difficulties that might arise peroperatively, for example a poorly dilated pupil would probably require a more senior surgeon to operate than in the case of a widely dilated one. The characteristics of the eyelids and orbit should also be assessed, as a deep-set eye with a narrow palpebral aperture will again necessitate a more experienced surgeon to be involved.

The experience of the surgeon involved in the procedure should also be taken into account when deciding which dilating drops to use as, although 2.5% and 10% phenylephrine both give good mydriasis preoperatively, a study by Duffin et al. showed that a 10% solution of phenylephrine was more effective than a 2.5% solution in maintaining mydriasis during extracapsular surgery.[3] They found that after nucleus expression the pupil area was 57% larger with the stronger concentration; this was particularly so in darkly pigmented irides, less so in moderately pigmented ones, and even less so in lightly pigmented irides. The mean blood pressure elevations were the same in both groups. Although this study involved extracapsular surgery, which is usually more traumatic for the eye and the iris in particular, if a junior surgeon is operating and the procedure takes longer than usual then consideration should be given to the above issue.

DILATING THE PUPIL

Phenylephrine 10% and cyclopentolate 1% are commonly used to dilate the pupil, but equally good results can be obtained using phenylephrine 2.5%, which may give a lower incidence of systemic side effects. The pupil size should be checked before the patient is transferred to theater, and any deficiency in dilatation should be reported to the operating surgeon. It is possible that this has been anticipated, for example in a patient with posterior synechiae, and perhaps the use of iris hooks to enlarge the pupil during surgery has been organized.

A large proportion of patients are able to walk to the operating theater. In a number of units, patients undergoing day surgery will not be required to change out of their outdoor clothing. Overshoes should be worn if outdoor shoes are kept on. The facility to transfer very elderly or infirm patients on a wheelchair or trolley bed should be available. In the case of a child, one or both parents should accompany the child to the anesthetic room. On arrival in the anesthetic room, the various checks should be made again; the theater staff need to be as convinced of the details of the patient and operation as the ward staff are. Five percent aqueous iodine can be instilled into the conjunctival sac at this point, and the patient prepared for administration of the anesthetic. Once patients are in the operating theater, they must be carefully positioned on the trolley or operating table so they are comfortable. Quite often, a pillow placed under the patient's knees makes him or her much more comfortable. If local anesthetic has been administered, a device for keeping the theater drapes off the patient's face should be placed on the operating table; this is usually in the form of a bar above the patient's face. The patient should be reassured that air or oxygen is delivered under the drapes during the procedure. It is extremely useful to have a member of the theater team holding the patient's hand so that she or he can reassure the patient and communicate with the patient and the surgeon. Patients can be instructed to squeeze this team member's hand if they are feeling any discomfort or wish to communicate with the surgeon. Some surgeons are happy for the patient to talk during the procedure, but others are not. Either way, the team member holding the patient's hand can often anticipate problems by being in tune with the patient's condition and feelings, which the surgeon may not be aware of, as the patient is covered up.

PREPARING THE OPERATING SITE

The skin around the eye is cleaned with 10% aqueous povidone–iodine solution. Four percent povidone–iodine has been found to be effective in reducing conjunctival commensals in a study by Barkana et al.[4]

Draping

Isolating the lashes and lid margins from the operating field is an important step in preventing entry of commensal organisms into the anterior chamber. A number of different methods of drape placement are available. Figure 4.1 shows the use of a thin cylindric instrument, such as a cotton bud or sheath from a syringe, to roll and evert the upper lid lashes out of the way. Another method is to ask the patient to look upward and, with the sticky part of the drape folded in half, use the drape itself to retract the upper lid lashes and then upfold the drape to isolate the lower lid lashes as

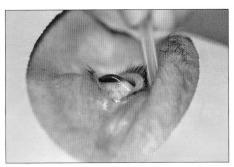

■ **FIGURE 4.1.** The upper lashes being everted using a cylindric cover from a hypodermic needle.

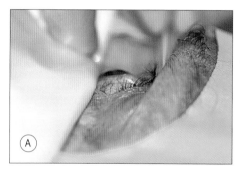

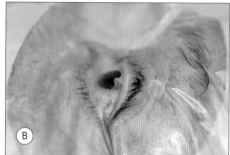

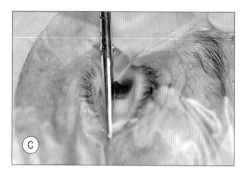

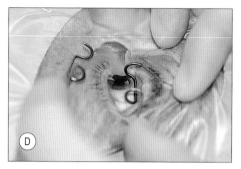

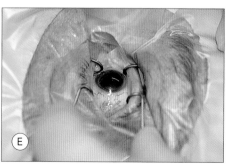

■ **FIGURE 4.2.** (**A**) The lashes of the lower lid are retracted using the folded sticky surface of the plastic drape. (**B**) The drape in position on the eye keeps both sets of lashes well everted. (**C**) Blunt-tipped scissors are used to incise the drape. (**D**) The speculum is inserted under the upper lid, carrying with it the plastic drape that wraps around the upper lid margin. (**E**) The same is done with the lower lid.

well (Fig. 4.2). A central incision is made in the drape horizontally in the midline between the two lids, and a relieving incision at the inner canthus inferiorly and superiorly can also be made. This allows the plastic drape to be folded over the edge of the lid into the inferior and superior conjunctival fornices. It is worth warning the patient that they may feel a speculum against the eyelid, which is probably not anesthetic. They otherwise worry that the eye itself may be sensitive during the procedure.

With the patient draped and the speculum in position between the lids, the operating microscope is bought into position. It is important that the surgeon has adjusted her or his chair to suit the height of the microscope; the height of the operating table can then be adjusted to suit the surgeon's sitting position (Fig. 4.3). Ideally, the surgeon

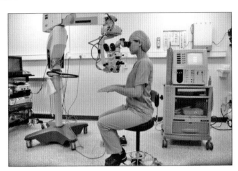

FIGURE 4.3. The ideal sitting position, with the surgeon comfortable on the stool, elbows held at approximately 90°, and the microscope adjusted to suit this position. The patient and operating table are then adjusted so that the surgeon can maintain this position in comfort throughout the procedure.

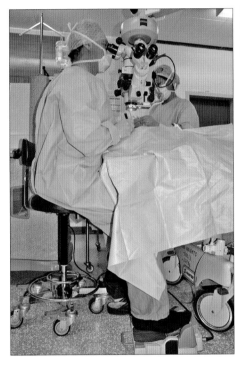

FIGURE 4.4. The surgeon at work with the feet comfortably positioned on the pedals; the patient and operating table have been positioned to suit his position.

should operate with the elbows bent at approximately 90°, and the feet comfortably placed on the microscope and phacoemulsification pedals (Fig. 4.4). If the incision for cataract surgery is placed temporally on the cornea and the surgeon is sitting at the patient's side, some operating tables or trolleys do not allow such easy access; this should be borne in mind when purchasing them. At this point, it should be checked that the image on the video monitor is in focus and centered, and that, if the procedure is being recorded, the recording device is started. It is also important to check that the patient is comfortable before beginning the procedure, and that the other members of the team are ready.

REFERENCES

1. Steinberg EP, Tielsch JM, Schein OD, et al. The VF 14: an index of functional impairment in patients with cataract. Arch Ophthalmol 1994; 112(5):630–638.

2. Lawrence DJ, Brogan C, Benjamin L, et al. Measuring the effectiveness of cataract surgery: the reliability and validity of a visual function outcomes instrument. Br J Ophthalmol 1999; 83(1):66–70.

3. Duffin RM, Pettit TH, Straatsma BR. 2.5% versus 10% phenylephrine in maintaining mydriasis during cataract surgery. Arch Ophthalmol 1983; 101(12):1903–1906.

4. Barkana Y, Almer Z, Segal O, et al. Reduction of conjunctival bacterial flora by povidone–iodine, ofloxacin and chlorhexidine in an outpatient setting. Acta Ophthalmol Scand 2005; 83(3):3603.

5 Wound placement and construction

Box 5.1 shows the large number of advantages of phaco-emulsification surgery over traditional extracapsular techniques. In order to maximize these advantages, the placement and structure of the wound into the eye must be carefully considered. With the advent of folding intraocular lens implants, the width of the phacoemulsification wound can be kept as small as 3 mm, and the surgically induced astigmatism may be negligible. However, incorrect placement and/or construction of the wound may cause significant problems with astigmatism, wound instability, and possibly even infection, thus negating a number of the stated advantages.

The principles of wound placement may relate to a number of factors. The further the wound is placed from the optical axis, the less surgically induced astigmatism will be present. Operating on the steep meridian of the cornea will tend to flatten it and will reduce any pre-existing astigmatism. This can be useful in trying to make the cornea more spherical, especially with the use of multifocal implants, which depend on corneal sphericity for maximum effect. Another important factor is pre-existing pathology, such as glaucoma. If filtering surgery is contemplated, then it is important not to interfere with the conjunctiva in the superior fornix, and so this may influence the chosen position of the wound. It is also important to consider whether a surgeon is right- or left-handed, for ease of access and wound placement may need to be shifted in order to avoid compounding pre-existing astigmatism with surgically induced changes.

BOX 5.1 Advantages of small-incision surgery over large-incision extracapsular techniques

- Less surgically induced astigmatism
- Faster visual rehabilitation
- Stronger wound
- Less endothelial cell loss
- No suture-related problems
- Reduced postoperative inflammation

SCLERAL TUNNEL INCISION

5.1

On the basis that the further away from the optical center of the eye an incision is made, the less astigmatic change is induced, scleral tunnels give a distinct advantage in keeping well away from the refractive surface of the eye. Traditional scleral tunnel incisions involve three distinct planes and two steps, and can be incredibly strong.

Figure 5.1 shows the construction of a scleral tunnel incision, both from the surgeon's view down the microscope and as corresponding diagrammatic side views. The conjunctiva is moved off the surface of the eye at the limbus, and a one-third scleral depth wound is made with a 15° blade. A crescent knife is then used to create a scleral pocket, which runs parallel to the surface of the sclera at one-third scleral depth; this is channeled forward approximately 1 mm into clear cornea. The third plane and second step is created with a preset-width slit knife. This is inserted into the scleral pocket initially parallel to the surface of the sclera, then the heel of the blade is raised so that the blade is parallel with the iris plane, and it is inserted into the anterior chamber. The full width of the blade must be used to ensure that the tunnel is the correct width for the phaco tip and infusion sleeve. The slit knife must be matched to the type and size of phaco needle and irrigating sleeve being used. This is to ensure a relatively watertight fit of the infusion sleeve and to allow some maneuverability of the phaco tip inside the eye. If an adequate width tunnel is not made, then pressure can occur on the infusion sleeve; this can restrict irrigation of fluid into the eye and diminish cooling of the phaco needle during emulsification. The scleral tunnel is usually begun around 2 mm behind the limbus, and therefore the tunnel usually ends up as being relatively square in shape when viewed down the microscope. This allows a relatively flat trajectory of the phaco needle into the eye and good maneuverability with very little distortion of the cornea. These two-step, three-plane wounds are very strong and will self-seal easily.

At the finish of the procedure, the conjunctiva must be replaced over the wound and can be held in place with a single 8/0 absorbable suture. Some surgeons use the subconjunctival injection in the conjunctival flap to try to reposition it, but not infrequently the flap will be relatively mobile and uncomfortable for the patient. Scleral tunnels can be useful in patients with poor endothelial function, for example from Fuchs endothelial dystrophy, as this form of wound probably leads to loss of fewer epithelial cells. Scleral tunnel incision can also be combined with trabeculectomy. Although initial reports of these combined sutureless phaco-trabeculectomies were promising,[1] there is increasing evidence that the pressure drop produced by these combined procedures may not be as great as that found with separate operations.

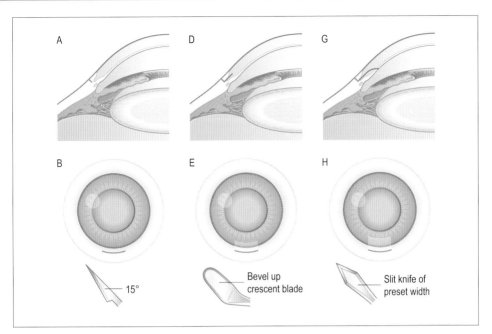

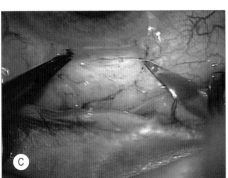

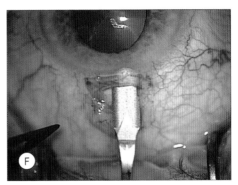

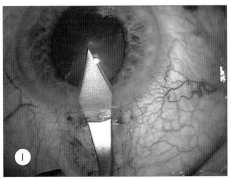

■ **FIGURE 5.1** (**A,B,C**) A surgeon's view and side view of the initial one-third thickness scleral groove being made, the conjunctival flap having been moved from the limbus. (**D,E,F**) The second stage of the procedure is a bevel up crescent blade used to create a scleral pocket. The pocket is roughly square and advanced into clear cornea, kept parallel to the surface of the eye. (**G,H,I**) Once the slit knife is entered into the pocket, initially with the same trajectory as the pocket was constructed, the heel of the blade is lifted and the blade inserted into the anterior chamber, parallel to the iris. This creates a two-step, three-plane wound.

CLEAR CORNEAL INCISION

The same principles apply for the construction of a clear corneal incision, but the wound is started just inside the limbus and the tunnel is kept much shorter, usually between 1 and 2 mm. If this is not done, then the tunnel length inhibits access to the superior part of the capsule when performing the capsulorrhexis. In addition, the angle of the phaco probe is much steeper into the eye with a long tunnel, and this can predispose to a phaco burn by constricting the infusion sleeve. The final disadvantage of a long phaco tunnel in the cornea is that the probe has to be introduced quite a long way into the eye to ensure that the infusion sleeve holes are in the anterior chamber and can provide irrigation. The tip of the needle will necessarily therefore be over halfway across the cataract before phacoemulsification can begin if this is the case. A short corneal tunnel is therefore in order.

The planes and steps of the tunnel construction can be the same, but a lot of surgeons miss out the formal pocket construction in the cornea and, having created an initial groove, will simply use the slit knife to create a small pocket into the stroma before changing direction with the blade and penetrating the anterior chamber. Indeed, another alternative is to miss out the formal groove altogether and simply use the slit knife to create a two-plane, one-stepped wound by pushing it into the stroma initially, parallel to the surface of the cornea, about 1 mm, and then lifting the heel of the blade upward and changing trajectory to enter the anterior chamber relatively parallel to the iris. These wounds are reasonably watertight and relatively strong. What is unacceptable is a forward-sloping wound in which the slit knife is simply plunged into the corneal and anterior chamber with no step and no change in plane. These wounds will often leak and be unstable, especially if they are enlarged to introduce an intraocular lens implant. Figure 5.2 shows construction of a corneal wound and demonstrates the two-plane, one-step wound, missing out the construction of a formal corneal pocket. A corneal wound may be necessary where an existing filtering bleb inhibits access to the sclera.

Some surgeons choose to gain access to the eye through a clear temporal corneal incision, on the basis that the cornea is horizontally oval, and that therefore the horizontal dimension of the cornea is longer than the vertical one. This means that a peripherally placed clear temporal corneal incision will be further away from the optical center than a superior one. This temporally placed incision can also give better access, especially with a deep-set eye, but there are also concerns about a slight increase in the risk of endophthalmitis for corneal incisions generally and temporal incisions especially.[2]

Taban et al. carried out a systematic review of the literature relating to endophthalmitis from 1963 to 2003.[3]

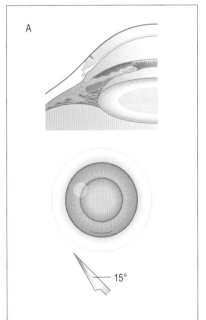

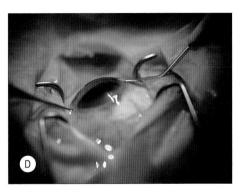

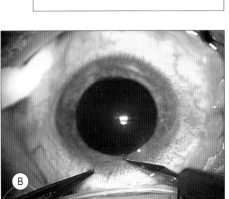

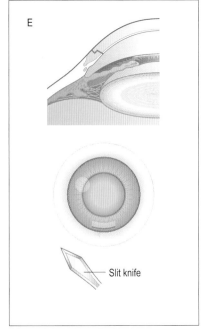

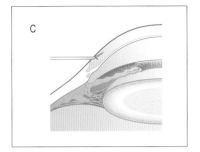

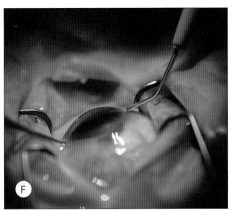

■ **FIGURE 5.2 (A–G)** Corneal wound construction. These steps are similar to those for a scleral tunnel but are often modified to miss out the formal formation of a pocket. A groove, as seen in (A), is still useful as a guide for centering the slit knife and also to provide the first step of the wound. Note the difference in angle of the blade between (**D**) and (**F**).

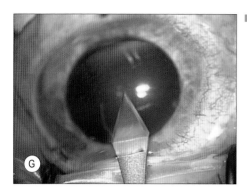

■ **FIGURE 5.2** (*con't*)

Interestingly, the incidence of acute endophthalmitis changed over time, with an increase since 2000 compared with previous decades. The rate of endophthalmitis was 0.265% in 2000–2003, 0.087% in the 1990s, 0.158% in the 1980s, and 0.327% during the 1970s. Endophthalmitis following clear corneal cataract extraction in the period 1992–2003 was 0.189%, compared with 0.074% for scleral incisions and 0.062% for limbal incisions. The researchers' conclusions from this systematic review were that the incidence of endophthalmitis associated with cataract extraction has increased over the past decade, and that this increase coincides temporarily with the development of sutureless clear corneal incisions. Of course, a systematic review such as this cannot necessarily link a cause and effect, and it may be that the period of time studied also coincided with many more people learning phacoemulsification and the cases taking longer.

From a practical point of view, when sutureless clear corneal incisions are made in any position of the cornea they are often enlarged to implant the intraocular lens. This enlargement is rarely measured; it is possible that the wounds are made much larger than expected, and this may lead to their instability. This might especially be so with temporal incisions, as the wound is inbetween the lids in the palpebral aperture and may be more prone to fish mouthing and allowing the contents of the tear film to be sucked into the eye postoperatively, for example if the eye is rubbed. All this is speculative but nevertheless is worthy of careful consideration when determining the site and size of the wound to be used, and there is some experimental evidence to suggest that entry of surface fluid does occur in the paper by Taban et al.[4]

ENLARGING THE WOUND

This is often necessary to introduce the intraocular lens, and the plane of enlargement should be as close to that of the original wound as possible. A slit knife or 15° blade can be used, and the amount of enlargement should be measured for consistent, repeatable accuracy for a given implant. By placing the cutting edge of the blade against one edge of the wound and cutting gently inward toward the center of the anterior chamber, a reliable cutting pressure can be maintained and reproduced. Figure 5.3 shows a corneal wound being enlarged.

ASTIGMATIC EFFECTS

Figure 5.4 shows the concept of an astigmatic funnel within which any horizontal incision will give the same degree of astigmatism. It can be seen from this that the more peripheral the incision, the less astigmatism is induced. Another way of saying this is that wider incisions can be

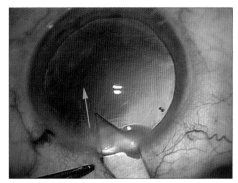

■ **FIGURE 5.3** A slit knife is used to enlarge the corneal wound. The arrow shows the direction of movement of the blade to ensure even enlargement of the inner and outer aspects of the wound.

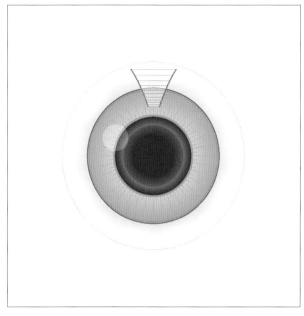

■ **FIGURE 5.4** The astigmatic funnel. Theoretically, any wound within this funnel shape will give identical astigmatism. It can be seen that a wound closer to the optical axis needs to be smaller than a wound further away for the same amount of surgically induced astigmatism.

Table 5.1 Astigmatic effects of different wounds

Wound type	Site	Wound width (mm)	Range of surgically induced astigmatism (diopters)
Scleral tunnel	Superior	3.2	0.2–1.0
incision	Oblique	5.5	0.6–1.5
Clear corneal	Superior	3.5	0.2–1.4
incision	Temporal	3.5	0.2–1.0

used in the sclera than in the cornea. Table 5.1 briefly summarizes the astigmatic effect according to incision length and position, as described by various authors. These various studies were done using very carefully measured wounds, and it is important to realize that wound enlargement, particularly for placement of an intraocular lens, is often done 'by eye' rather than measured. It is therefore quite possible to induce much larger amounts of astigmatism than one anticipates, and that this effect can be variable from case to case if the wounds are not measured.

Preoperative keratometry will confirm corneal dimensions and give a good guide to what may need to be done intraoperatively to correct astigmatism. More importantly, it will guide the surgeon where not to place the wound in order to induce larger amounts of astigmatism. Most patients develop against the rule astigmatism with age, which means that the horizontal meridian is steeper; therefore a temporally placed incision will reduce this astigmatism. If this fact is missed, and patients do indeed have against the rule astigmatism preoperatively and the wound is placed superiorly, it is possible to give them 1 or 2 diopters of surgically induced astigmatism, which, added to their own, may relatively easily cause 4 or 5 diopters of postoperative astigmatism. This can be quite difficult to manage and may require further surgery in the form of astigmatic keratotomy.

Careful preoperative planning is therefore essential to avoid astigmatic surprises, as it is clear that the approach of having one set incision site and size is not appropriate for all patients. It will sometimes be necessary to operate from the temporal side, sometimes from the superior aspect, and, depending on the patient's requirements, a scleral or a corneal incision may be required. It is important to learn all these techniques in order to give the patient the maximum benefit from their small incision surgery.

If the wound is enlarged to more than about 4 mm in width, then it is likely that it will be less stable, and a simple cross-stitch can be placed in the wound to close it securely. This is shown in Figure 5.5; by starting the suture in the depth of the wound and completing in the opposite side of the wound, the knot will automatically be buried. If a phaco burn has occurred, it is important not to try to oppose the edges of the wound, but simply to close them in

5.4

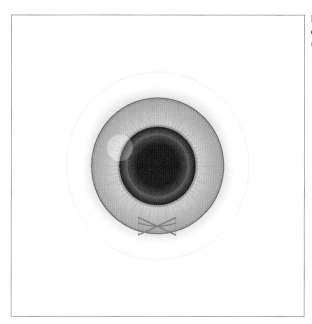

■ **FIGURE 5.5** An infinity or cross-suture used to close an unstable phaco wound.

an anteroposterior direction, otherwise large amounts of astigmatism can be induced. The burn causes tissue shrinkage, and the anterior lip of the wound will contract away from its fellow posterior lip; trying to pull the one up to meet the other will cause a major shift in corneal steepness.

If the wound is relatively stable, then simple stromal hydration can be used to temporarily swell the edges of the wound to ensure closure while the patient is transferred off the operating table and back to the recovery area. Figure 5.6 shows stromal hydration taking place.

THE SIDE PORT

The side port should be made with a 15° blade, and should be made just big enough to admit the second instrument into the anterior chamber. It is a useful maneuver to hold the main wound groove with the notched forceps and to position the side port blade where it is comfortable in relation to the hand that will be holding the phaco probe (Fig. 5.7). Side ports are made at the limbus, roughly parallel to the iris plane and small enough to be self-sealing. Some surgeons prefer to use a Simcoe type of cannula to remove the soft lens matter during the irrigation–aspiration phase of the procedure. If this is the case, the side port used for this should be enlarged at that point in the procedure, rather than at the beginning. This is because a large side port will allow excess fluid to escape from the anterior chamber, and create anterior chamber instability and flutter. A second side port at a similar angle from, but on the other side to, the main wound can be useful, for example to

5.5

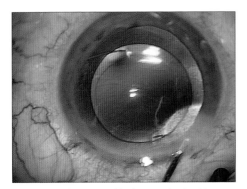

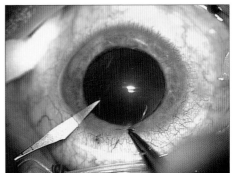

■ **FIGURE 5.6** Stromal hydration obtained by placing the cannula against the medial and lateral walls of the wound and injecting balanced salt solution into the stroma.

■ **FIGURE 5.7** Construction of the side port. The initial groove, made with a 15° blade, is held with a pair of notched forceps to give the surgeon tactile feedback of roughly where the phaco probe will be held with the right hand. The side port wound is made where it is comfortable with respect to this groove.

access the capsular flap during capsulorrhexis. It is useful to make the side port at the limbus, as it is often possible to detect its position from a small amount of bleeding that occurs from the limbal arcades. Another useful tip is to mark the position of the side port with gentian violet. This technique can also be used for marking the position of paracentesis sites used for iris hooks.

REFERENCES

1. Kownacki JD, Artaria LG. Sutureless phaco-trabeculectomy. Interim results. Klin Monatsbl Augenheilkd 2000; 216(5):250–255.
2. Taban M, Behrens A, Newcomb RL, et al. Acute endophthalmitis following cataract surgery: a systemic review of the literature. Arch Ophthalmol 2005; 123(5):613–620.
3. Taban M, Behrens A, Newcombe RL, et al. Acute endophthalmitis following cataract surgery: a systematic review of the literature. Arch Ophthalmol 2005; 123(5):613–620.
4. Taban M, Sarayba MA, Ignacia TS, et al. Ingress of India ink into the anterior chamber through sutureless clear corneal cataract wounds. Arch Ophthalmol 2005; 123(5):643–648.

6 Viscoelastics

A viscoelastic, as its name suggests, has properties of both viscosity and elasticity. True viscoelastics also exhibit pseudoplastic behavior, which means that they change their viscosity as they move faster. This enables very viscous agents to be injected down very fine cannulae, as they shear-thin or become less viscous as they move faster down the small cannula. They have become indispensable as a soft surgical tool for moving tissues gently, allowing movement of instruments in the anterior chamber, maintaining space, and in some cases providing some hemostatic properties. One of the main functions is endothelial protection. Early studies demonstrated that the use of viscoelastics reduced endothelial cell loss during extracapsular surgery.

TYPES OF VISCOELASTIC

Viscoelastics can be broadly divided into dispersive, cohesive, and adaptive. These particular properties relate to the molecule size, the negative charge on the molecule, and the extent to which the tertiary structure is folded. Two naturally occurring substances, sodium hyaluronate and chondroitin sulfate, are commonly found in surgical viscoelastics. Plant-derived hydroxypropylmethylcellulose (HPMC) is also used but exhibits much lower pseudoplastic behavior than the other two do. Hyaluronic acid binding sites have also been found on the endothelial cells. It is thought that sodium hyaluronate can bind to these cells during surgery, and perhaps produce a biolayer that persists postoperatively and may protect against postoperative inflammation.

DISPERSIVE VISCOELASTICS

Dispersive viscoelastics are so called because the molecule disperses easily and has a low viscosity. These agents are less easily removed from the eye, as the molecules tend not to stick together, but they are very useful agents for coating instruments and for endothelial protection. Examples of dispersive agents are Viscoat (Alcon), which is a mixture of sodium hyaluronate and chondroitin sulfate, and Occucoat, which is HPMC. Both these substances have a low resting viscosity.

COHESIVE VISCOELASTICS

Examples of these are Healon (AMO), Provisc (Alcon), and Healon GV (greater viscosity) (AMO), all of which have a resting shear rate of > 100 000. These cohesive agents are very good at forming and maintaining surgical spaces, and are relatively easy to remove by aspiration because the molecules tend to stick together.

VISCOADAPTIVE

The relatively newly developed Healon 5 has a molecular weight of 5 million Daltons, and its tertiary structure gives it properties somewhere between those of a dispersive and a cohesive viscoelastic. It is excellent at maintaining space and allowing safe maneuverability of surgical instruments, but is also relatively easy to remove, as a molecule can be divided into cohesive elements that can be aspirated safely. The technique of removal for this agent is known as the 'rock and roll' technique, and involves moving the irrigation–aspiration cannula from side to side to facilitate removal of the agent.

While there are studies demonstrating that HPMC-type molecules seem to protect endothelium as well as sodium hyaluronate–based agents do,[1] there are also studies demonstrating that, with very hard nuclei, there is greater protection against cell loss using specific techniques, such as the soft-shell technique.[2] The soft-shell technique involves injecting a dispersive viscoelastic up against the cornea and a cohesive viscoelastic underneath it, against the lens. The dispersive agent forms a soft shell against the endothelium and protects it, even if the more cohesive viscoelastic, which is in the surgical field, comes out during phacoemulsification (Fig. 6.1). Figure 6.2 shows a graph of viscosity versus shear rate for a number of agents. It demonstrates clearly that the more viscous agents have a greater change in viscosity with increasing shear rate. This makes the more viscous agents much safer to use for inexperienced surgeons, or when unexpected things may occur during surgery, such as the collapse of a chamber. It is therefore important that trainees use substances that exhibit greater pseudoplastic properties; for this reason, the routine use of HPMC for trainee surgeons is not sensible.

VISCOELASTIC USE IN CATARACT SURGERY

Certain points of the procedure mandate the use of a good pseudoplastic viscoelastic. The first of these is the capsulorrhexis when a deep, full chamber is necessary to complete the maneuver safely. Details of this are found in Chapter 7. Lens implantation is another stage that requires a full and deep chamber as well as maintenance of the surgical space to allow safe unfolding of the implant without injuring the endothelium.

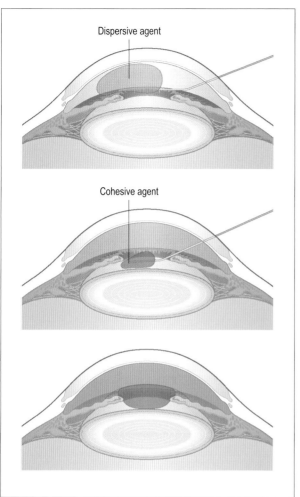

■ **FIGURE 6.1** The soft-shell technique. A coating, or shell, of dispersive viscoelastic is injected into the anterior chamber. A cohesive viscoelastic is then injected underneath this, against the surface of the lens. This provides protection, even during phacoemulsification, as the cohesive viscoelastic is less easily removed by the phaco probe.

Adequate removal of the viscoelastic is important to prevent intraocular pressure rise postoperatively and also other complications, such as distension of the capsular bag, which can cause a myopic shift or even acute angle closure glaucoma. Removal of viscoelastic from behind the implant may be necessary by placing the irrigation–aspiration cannula posterior to the implant. HPMC is very useful for coating the cornea during surgery, as it provides a smooth optical surface that is fairly stable; this is particularly useful if an assistant is not present to apply drops on to the cornea during surgery.

SUMMARY

Viscoelastics are indispensable soft surgical tools that have made intraocular surgery much safer and some maneuvers much easier. They should be used routinely for training, to

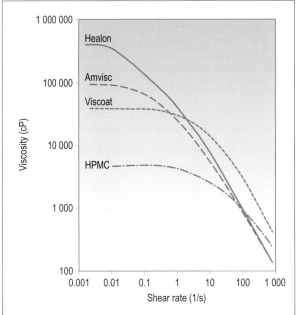

FIGURE 6.2 Viscosity plotted against shear rate for a number of viscoelastic substances. It can be seen that some are better than others at changing their viscosity; these are the more pseudoplastic substances.

provide a safe intraocular environment for the trainee and prevent surprises. They should be thoroughly removed from the eye at the end of surgery.

REFERENCES

1. Lane SS, Naylor DW, Kullerstrand LJ, et al. Prospective comparison of the effects of Occucoat, Viscoat and Healon on intraocular pressure and endothelial cell loss. J Cataract Refract Surg 1991; 17(1):21–26.

2. Kim H, Joo CK. Efficacy of the soft-shell technique using Viscoat and Hyal-2000. J Cataract Refract Surg 2004; 30(11):2366–2370.

7 Capsulorrhexis and capsule problems

Brian Little

CAPSULORRHEXIS

Background

Like many significant innovations in surgery, the technique of capsulorrhexis seems so glaringly obvious in retrospect that many of us cannot quite believe we never thought of it ourselves. But we definitely did not, and so must remain gratefully and eternally indebted to Neuhann and Gimbel, who did.[1,2]

Although continuous curvilinear capsulorrhexis (CCC) was originally developed for use in phacoemulsification surgery, for which it has now been universally adopted, it is also gaining widespread popularity in non-phaco sutureless cataract surgery in developing countries, simply because it is without equal as the most reliable way of creating a secure and resilient opening in the anterior lens capsule (Dr. Albrecht Hennig, Lahan Eye Hospital, Nepal, personal communication).

Although simple in theory, many experienced surgeons still consider the rhexis to be the single most technically challenging step of phaco to get right every time. The fact that it is so globally popular despite this challenge is testimony to the significant functional advantages that it offers. Safe endocapsular phaco has become possible only because of it.

The three Cs of the abbreviation also conveniently represent the three principal technical challenges posed by the rhexis: it needs to be circular, central, and the correct size.

This chapter is intended to provide you with a solid and practical foundation on which to build the surgical skills that will enable you to achieve these aims. With additional supervised experience and repeated practice, you will, over time, master the challenges of this undeniably important step of modern cataract surgery, which in practice occupies only about 1 minute out of the life of an experienced phaco surgeon.

Instruments

The CCC procedure was first performed using the cheapest microsurgical instrument known to us: a bent hypodermic needle (see Gimbel and Neuhann 1991[2]). Although it has its limitations, a custom-shaped or preformed cystotome is still very popular today as the instrument of choice for many surgeons. Most use a 25-gauge needle, because the finer

27-gauge can be a little too flexible for optimal control of the tear. The advantages of a needle (apart from being so cheap and with no repair bills) come from its small size and maneuverability: it can be used through a side port and causes minimal wound distortion. This reduces the all-important risk of chamber collapse from loss of viscoelastic. Its only disadvantage is that you are obliged to press downward on to the capsule in order to gain any traction; this reduces the degrees of freedom for directional control of the tear.

Next up the evolutionary scale come the Utrata or parallel-action capsulorrhexis forceps (Fig. 7.1). Although a significant innovation, in that they allow you to apply traction in any chosen direction, the earlier models were relatively bulky, causing wound gape and frequent chamber collapse as well as obscuring the view of the tear under their tips. Finer-gauge versions have improved matters a little, but their parallel mode of action still has the inherent disadvantage that the portion of the shafts within the tunnel will always be open wider than the tips of the jaws, and thus will tend to cause wound gape and distortion.

These issues inspired the development of scissor-action or cross-action forceps with finer shafts and les acutely angled jaws (Fig. 7.2). The cross-action mechanism gives more sensitive control of the opening and closing of the jaws through mechanical advantage, and the low-profile hinge results in less wound gape (Inamura D&K). The softer angulation of the jaws also allows direct visibility of their tips and the underlying capsule.

Coaxial forceps have been used routinely by vitreoretinal surgeons for many years but have only more recently attracted the attention of frustrated bimanual microincision phaco surgeons seeking an alternative to the needle as their hitherto only option for capsulorrhexis (Fig. 7.3). This has driven the development and refinement of coaxial forceps for performing capsulorrhexis. They offer exquisite control and maneuverability, but at an equally exquisite cost. They also require careful washing and maintenance, otherwise trapped viscoelastic gets autoclaved inside the

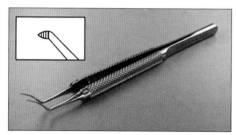

■ **FIGURE 7.1.** Utrata-style uncrossed or parallel-action capsulorrhexis forceps. (Courtesy of Duckworth & Kent.)

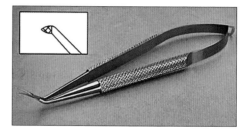

■ **FIGURE 7.2.** Cross-action Inamura-style capsulorrhexis forceps. (Courtesy of Duckworth & Kent.)

lumen, which rapidly renders them useless except as a costly Christmas tree decoration.

The last instrument worthy of mention is Kloti radio-frequency diathermy, which enjoyed a brief period of cele-brity as a foolproof method for anterior capsulotomy in dense adult cataracts with little or no red reflex, and in pediatric cataracts in which the highly elastic capsule is notoriously difficult to tear accurately. Its usefulness has been largely superseded by the use of capsular dyes to visualize the anterior capsule, and the recognition of the more brittle edge of the rhexis created with this technique.[2]

In practice, your choice of instrument is one of personal preference. However, it behoves all surgeons to develop the capacity for adaptability. Adaptability allows us to move effortlessly between a number of alternative options when the situation we are faced with demands it. Capsulorrhexis similarly requires us to be able to use a needle and forceps with equal facility, as neither of them alone is adequate for all situations. If, in addition, you can learn to use them in either hand, and also tear the capsule both clockwise and counterclockwise, then you are likely to be able to straddle most of the hurdles that performing capsulorrhexis can throw in your path. This level of control gives you choice, and choice gives you adaptability.

CAPSULORRHEXIS TECHNIQUE

Like every step in phaco, the devil is in the detail, and this is particularly true when performing capsulorrhexis. Careful attention is needed to the finer points of the technique, because small errors at this stage can result in significant complications later on.

Preparation

Before you even think about starting the rhexis, you need to begin with good preparation. Remember the universally ap-plicable five Ps: proper preparation prevents poor perform-ance. This important preparatory phase is easily overlooked

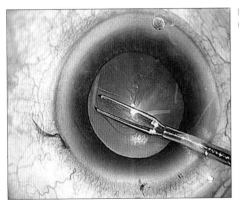

■ **FIGURE 7.3.** Coaxial capsulorrhexis forceps. (Courtesy of B.C. Little.)

in the rush to get on with the surgery. (Remember *proper preparation*.) It starts with the selection of easy eyes if you are a beginner. The ideal eye for a novice is one that has a shallow orbit, easily retracted lids, good akinesia and anesthesia, a clear cornea, a deep chamber, a well-dilated pupil, and a good red reflex. If you can tick all these boxes, then you are off to a good start. (Remember *easy eyes*.)

Next, you need to ensure that the patient is comfortable and well positioned so that the eye is optimally accessible, with good coaxial illumination. Before you start the surgery, try covering the cornea with methylcellulose and let it spread out evenly. You will be surprised just how much this improves visibility, and it needs only a very occasional top up during surgery.

The incisions come next. Even if you normally use just one side port, it can be very helpful indeed to routinely make two. Position them either side of the main incision and separated by between 90 and 120°. This costs you absolutely nothing but allows you universal access from either side with a cystotome. Should you need such access later on, everything is already prepared for you.

If you favor a superior approach then, before you start, make sure that the speculum is positioned so that the ends of the open upper blade are either side of the tunnel to avoid snagging the forceps or needle on the speculum once your instrument is inside the eye. The stage is now set.

First and foremost, you must completely fill the chamber with viscoelastic. Try to backfill with a continuous wave rather than a discontinuous 'worm' that can leave lacunae of trapped aqueous. Most surgeons prefer to use a cohesive agent, because these are generally better retained in the eye during capsulorrhexis. The cohesive properties of Healon 5 are quite outstanding in this respect, and it provides an extraordinarily stable chamber. It is slightly more problematic to completely remove, but this is a small price to pay for its positive benefits. These become particularly apparent with challenging cases such as a shallow chamber, a small pupil, or an intumescent cataract. It is not essential, but it can be particularly helpful.

The purpose of the viscoelastic is to pressurize the anterior chamber, and thereby tamponade the forward movement of the lens that is caused by positive vitreous pressure from behind. The lens capsule is an elastic membrane that is held in place by the zonules attached around its equator. You can appreciate that any forward movement of the lens will place the anterior capsule under additional tension when the zonules are put on stretch. If you tear the anterior capsule in this state of heightened tension, then the tear will tend to rip out toward the equator along the tension vectors. This is why it is absolutely imperative that the chamber should remain as full as possible at all times during the capsulorrhexis. Any partial chamber collapse means forward movement of the lens and likely extension of the tear toward the equator. The viscoelastic pushes back the lens, flattens the anterior capsule, and neutralizes the tension, thereby reducing the tendency of the tear to extend toward the equator. So the first article of faith is at all times to keep the chamber full of viscoelastic. (Remember *chock-full chamber*.) This is probably the single most important tip to help you keep control of the tear and prevent it escaping peripherally. To start with, discipline yourself to stop every 90° and refill the chamber even if you do not think you need to: you will be surprised at how much has escaped undetected. In an eye with a shallow chamber or more positive vitreous pressure, you may well need to refill even more often than this. (Remember *regular refills*.)

Performing the capsulorrhexis

Now for the rhexis itself. First, adjust the zoom on the microscope so that the cornea fills between half and two-thirds of the field, and then focus down on to the capsule.

The first step is to initiate the tear. This can be done in a number of ways: with the keratome (as a follow-through after the main incision), with a cystotome needle, or with the closed points of the capsulorrhexis forceps or with them open using just one jaw to puncture the capsule. Whichever method you choose, the aim is to perforate the capsule just proximal to the center. The initial tear then needs to be converted into a flap. This can be done either by pushing the instrument forward to form a small triangular flap, or alternatively by extending the tear radially and then lifting the instrument forward from under the capsule toward the cornea. This forces the end of the tear to break out circumferentially and form a flap.

As soon as you have made this flap, then fold it over and grasp the free peripheral edge close to the apex of the tear and, keeping it as flat as possible in the plane of the capsule, propagate the tear parallel to the pupil margin. (Remember *flat flap*.)

Until you are more experienced, you should make just small tears and frequently go back and regrasp the flap at the apex. You may take eight or more sectors to begin with, but with experience this will come down to three or four. (Remember *tiny tears*.)

To avoid wound distortion and unwanted eye movement from transmitted instrument movement, you must learn to allow your instrument to 'float' in the wound, which itself should act as a neutral pivot or fulcrum for rotation of your instrument. (Remember *float and pivot*.)

The force vector that tears the capsule in the intended direction is the resolution of two components: a central element and a circumferential element. You need to appreciate that the required central vector of the traction becomes greater as the rhexis progresses (Fig. 7.4). So, for the final few degrees, you will need to pull the flap almost completely centrally, perpendicular to the circumferential

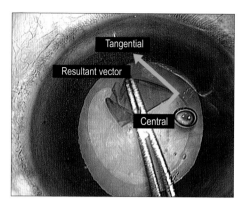

■ **FIGURE 7.4.** The resolution of central and tangential vector forces to tear the capsule circumferentially. (Courtesy of B.C. Little.)

direction of the tear. Some surgeons appreciate this issue of vector resolution much more intuitively than others, but everyone is capable of learning it. It is impossible to teach from a book and is much easier to understand in practice. Another fact to appreciate regarding the forces involved is that you get no tangible force feedback as the capsule tears, i.e. capsulorrhexis is entirely visually guided.

Making it the right size

If you have managed to control the tear and keep it parallel to and a fixed distance from the pupil margin, then your rhexis should fulfill two of the three Cs by being central and circular. It may not, however, fulfil the criterion of the third C, which is correct size. This is the most difficult one to get consistently right, and it is an inexact science. Have you ever seen any surgeon actually measure a capsulorrhexis or use a template?

As a novice, and often well beyond, the surgeon is frequently too preoccupied with averting disaster to worry about the size of the rhexis, which is most commonly undersized from being overcautious. Preoccupation with size is the preserve of the experienced surgeon with sufficient confidence and skill to control it. If you aim for a diameter of 5 mm, this will give you an edge overlap of 0.25 mm for a 5.5-mm optic and 0.5 mm for a 6-mm optic. Around 4 mm is the lower acceptable limit for the rhexis diameter; below this, the risk increases of complications such as capsule block, edge tear, and postoperative capsular phimosis. The concentric overlap of the rhexis, combined with a square-edged optic, appears to provide a mechanical barrier to lens epithelial cell migration across the posterior capsule, and thereby reduce the incidence of posterior lens capsule opacification (Dr. Albrecht Hennig, personal communication).

So how can you reliably judge the 5-mm diameter that you need? Well, you have to resist the obvious temptation to use the pupil as your reference, because its diameter is so variable. However, in contrast, the vertical diameter of the cornea is fairly fixed at around 10 mm, so you can use this as your reference. Think of the cornea as the optic disk and the rhexis as the cup, and mentally image a 0.5 cup:disk ratio. This should help you to get within the right range, but only surgical experience will refine and hone your judgment.

The subincisional sector

The subincisional part of the rhexis is the most awkward sector to keep under control because of wound distortion, mechanical discomfort, and instrumental obscuration of the tear. The easiest part of the rhexis is the first 90° from whatever point you start. So why not start with the subincisional sector first and turn the most difficult part into the easiest part? This sounds disarmingly simple, but it really does work. However, in practice, it is counterintuitive and requires the self-discipline to withstand the temptation to tread the path of least resistance and begin the rhexis diametrically opposite the main incision or obliquely off to one side. (Remember *start subincisionally.*)

If you are using forceps, then here is a specific technique that will help you to negotiate the subincisional sector with considerable success and reduced stress. It is described here for a counterclockwise tear. The idea in principle is to complete this sector by means of a controlled and continuous tear without having to release and regrasp the flap, as this so often leads to loss of control. Do this by terminating the previous tear just before you reach the left-hand edge of the incision. Begin with the forceps resting against the left side of the incision, and grasp the free edge of the flap as peripherally as you can. Slide the closed forceps over to the right side of the incision to tear the flap across its width. Now, using this edge of the incision as a pivot, rotate the closed forceps clockwise, then push them centrally and circumferentially to propagate the tear around and under the right-hand end of the incision. These movements of the forceps divide into three stages that, with practice, will merge fairly fluently into one: straight across, pivot clockwise, and push and continue around.

If you get stuck and are having difficulty controlling the subincisional tear, then stop, refill the chamber, and, if you are not already using one, swap to a needle cystotome mounted on the viscoelastic syringe and reenter the eye through one or other of the side ports. You get a much better view and can pull the flap around via one of them, push it around via the other, or do a bit of both. This is a particularly useful approach if the flap is long and prolapsing into the tunnel, carried by the flow of viscoelastic. It can be swept back into the eye from either side port. If it is being a persistent nuisance, then simply cut off the excess and continue.

As an aide-memoire, the important principles for successful capsulorrhexis are summarized as eight (mostly) alliterative guidelines in Box 7.1.

> **BOX 7.1 Capsulorrhexis guidelines**
> - Easy eyes
> - Proper preparation
> - Chock-full chamber
> - Float and pivot
> - Start subincisionally
> - Regular refills
> - Flat flap
> - Tiny tears

Summary

Probably the most important 60 seconds of any phaco operation is the time spent creating a central and circular rhexis of the correct size. It sets the stage for the rest of the operation. The secret to success lies in attention to detail. You must understand the way in which vector forces interact to control the direction of the tear, together with the utmost importance of maintaining at all times a deep chamber filled with viscoelastic. If you put this into practice, then you are likely to maintain the integrity of the anterior capsule and minimize the risk of potentially sight-threatening complications that can result from its loss.

CAPSULE PROBLEMS AND COMPLICATIONS

7.1

The main problems encountered during the rhexis are summarized in Table 7.1. This includes their causes, consequences, and suggested practical solutions.

There is one of these complications above all others that warrants more detailed discussion because of its particular importance, and that complication is a radial tear-out (Fig. 7.5). In the hands of an experienced surgeon, you can expect an incidence of less than 1%. When you consider that the adult anterior capsule is only 10–15 μm thick and that it becomes less elastic with age, it then seems surprising that the incidence is not higher. We can describe it as a radial extension of the capsulorrhexis tear. This gives an acronym (RECT) that phonetically describes its potential effect (i.e. wrecked) on the surgical outcome.

Your best strategy is obviously prevention in the first place, but when you have to deal with this complication, which is inevitable, then you need to deploy a clear escape plan with the primary objective of damage limitation.

Prevention first (Box 7.2). You need to appreciate the risk factors that increase the likelihood of a RECT so that you can anticipate, recognize, and as far as possible neutralize them. The commonest risk factor by a long way is chamber shallowing from loss of viscoelastic. This often goes unnoticed because:

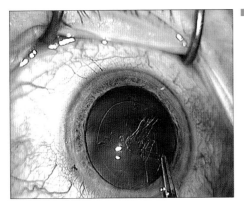

■ **FIGURE 7.5** Radial tear-out.

BOX 7.2 Avoiding radial tear-out
- Chock-full chamber
- Regular refills
- Flat flaps
- Tiny tears

- it happens slowly,
- you need to lose only a very small volume, and
- the surgeon's attention is focused 100% at the sharp end of the chosen instrument.

The need to keep the chamber filled throughout the rhexis should somehow be ingrained compulsorily either at birth or on admission to a residency program as a reverberating neural circuit in the brainstem of every eye surgeon. It should kick in as a pavlovian reflex at the earliest sign of trouble, or preferably just before. If, from the start, you routinely refill the chamber after each 90–120° sector of the rhexis, then this habit will become instilled at an early stage of your surgical development, thereby reducing to a minimum the risk of a tear-out (remember *regular refills*).

If chamber collapse is persistent despite such care, then you need to eliminate other possible causes. External pressure can arise from a number of sources (Box 7.3):

- the speculum (especially the non-adjustable thick-gauge wire type, Fig. 7.6), which may need to be loosened or preferably replaced with an adjustable type;
- lid tension from squeezing under topical anesthesia or from a particularly narrow interpalpebral fissure; and
- orbital tension from volume of local anesthetic.

Rare causes that you need to remain alert to are an intraoperative orbital hemorrhage and a suprachoroidal hemorrhage, which both cause aggressive and intractable shallowing.

TABLE 7.1 Capsule problems and complications during capsulorrhexis

Problem	Cause	Consequence	Solution
Poor visibility	Corneal scarring, pterygium, or edema.	Poor control of rhexis through reduced visibility. Risk of tear-out.	Optimize coaxial illumination. Use capsular dye. Methylcellulose on cornea.
Reduced red reflex	Dense or white cataract, small pupil.	Lost control of rhexis with risk of tear-out.	Capsular dye. Pupil enlargement.
Collapsing chamber	Positive pressure from vitreous or external origin: speculum pressure, drape tension, retrobulbar hemorrhage. Rarely suprachoroidal hemorrhage.	High risk of peripheral tear-out.	Eliminate external causes. Use Healon 5. Swap from main incision and use needle via side ports.
Loss of view of tear during rhexis	Disturbance of underlying cortex.	High risk of radial tear or peripheral tear-out.	Stop immediately. Refill with viscoelastic. Inject capsular dye to visualize tear.
Anterior capsule plaques	Previous blunt trauma. Calcified variety associated with dense, white, or hypermature cataracts.	–	Impossible to tear through tough plaques. Tear around them or cut through with scissors.
Small rhexis	Most commonly results from having a small pupil. Next is surgical inexperience.	High risk of capsule block during hydrodissection and edge tear from phaco tip or second instrument.	If in doubt, then enlarge it. Initiate with semitangential cut using capsule scissors and continue with forceps.

TABLE 7.1 (cont'd)

Problem	Cause	Consequence	Solution
Diaphanous friable capsule	Very elderly, mature cataracts, pseudoexfoliation.	Fragmentation of flap. Extremely delicate and easy to tear out.	The key to control is anticipation. Tear only small segments each time. Healon 5 is particularly useful for flap stabilization.
Double-layered capsule	Capsular schisis. Usually in elderly patients.	Disconcerting but no real danger. Rare but unavoidable.	May need separate rhexis for each layer.
Small radial tear or arrowhead notch.	Inadvertent damage from needle point. Residual notch from inside-out versus outside-in completion of rhexis.	Dangerous only if unseen. Almost inevitable peripheral extension later on.	If suspected, then stop and zoom in. Add capsular dye if poor visibility. Needs to be rounded off, producing scalloped out-pocket of rhexis.
Radial extension of capsulorrhexis tear	Centrifugal force vector. Usually resulting from chamber shallowing, occasionally due to surgeon error or intumescent lens.	High risk of wraparound tear and dropped nucleus.	Stop immediately. Refill with viscoelastic. Visualize apex of tear with or without dye. Attempt retrieval. Irretrievable once far into the zonules. Complete the rhexis with new cut from opposite direction.
Diametric split across anterior capsule (Argentine flag sign)	Intumescent lens with high capsular tension.	Unsafe for endocapsular phaco. High risk of wraparound tear and dropped nucleus.	Reduce risk by first overfilling chamber with viscoelastic to flatten the anterior lens. Then try initial capsule decompression via central perforation to release liquefied cortex.

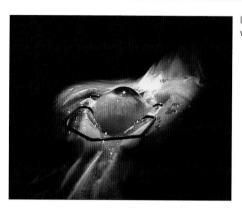

■ **FIGURE 7.6** Non-adjustable thick-gauge wire–type speculum.

BOX 7.3 Sources of external pressure
- Speculum
- Lid squeezing
- Narrow interpalpebral fissure
- Large volume of local anesthetic
- Intraoperative orbital hemorrhage

The rhexis can still tear out peripherally even in the presence of a deep chamber if the flap is lifted forward toward the cornea. Application of such vertical traction is only possible using forceps and is appropriate when you want to increase the radius of the tear, but if applied inappropriately is guaranteed absolutely without fail to rip it out toward the equator. To avoid this, keep the flap folded down flat against the underlying capsule at all times when propagating the tear (recall *flat flap*). The second point to note that will help you maintain directional control of the tear is to keep hold of the free edge of the flap as close as possible to the origin of the tear. This is achieved by tearing only a small segment at a time and frequently regrasping the flap back at its origin (remember *tiny tears*).

Now to outline the surgical options alluded to earlier that will help you manage a RECT when it happens and help to limit the damage (Box 7.4). First and foremost you must, at the earliest sign of trouble, avoid the cardinal sin of denial; do not be panicked into rushing ahead and trying to quickly finish the rhexis before it gets any worse. You should stay calm, stop immediately, and refill the chamber with viscoelastic. In general, those surgeons who have the insight to recognize the early signs of impending disaster and the self-discipline to take early evasive action when they are running into trouble (rather than after they have run into it) will avoid being sucked into the vortex generated by the downwardly spiralling cascade of surgical doom. As a consequence, they will get better results and

BOX 7.4 Managing radial tear-out

- Do not deny it.
- Stop and refill.
- Do not let the chamber collapse.
- Assess the extent.
- Iris retraction or hooks.
- 'Unfolded flap' retrieval technique.
- Alternative strategies if unsuccessful.

fewer complications. The ability to exercise this level of humility and self-discipline is a rare quality but an invaluable one for avoiding complications in general.

Having stopped and refilled the chamber, you now need to calmly assess the peripheral extent of the tear. In the ideal scenario, you will have stopped before it has run out too far and then found that deepening the chamber has adequately redilated the pupil to reveal the apex of the tear. You can now start breathing again and carry on where you left off. You probably just need to redirect the tear more centrally. In this case, the only penalty you pay in the end is the mainly cosmetic one of a pear-shaped or keyhole-shaped rhexis (Fig. 7.7).

Unfortunately, a RECT often unzips fairly rapidly and ends up in the zonules before the synaptic delays in the pathway of your escape reflex have allowed you to release the flap. Once into the zonules, retrieval of the tear becomes more difficult but by no means impossible. When you consider the local anatomy, you will realize that the tear does not have to travel out very far to reach the zonules (Fig. 7.8). The average diameter of the crystalline lens is 10.5 mm, and the insertion zone of the anterior zonules extends over a peripheral ring whose central edge

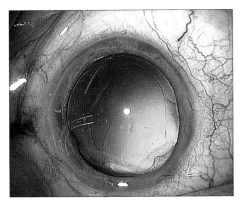

■ **FIGURE 7.7** Pear-shaped or keyhole-shaped rhexis.

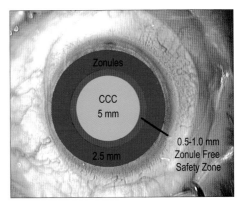

■ **FIGURE 7.8** Tear reaching the zonules.

lies 2.5 mm from the equator. This leaves a guaranteed zonule-free and rhexis-friendly central zone of only 5.5 mm in diameter, and you are aiming for a 5-mm rhexis—not a lot of room for error and only surprising that we do not end up in the zonules more often than we do.

Once the tear involves the zonules, your options are limited but clear. First, you need to have a good view of the leading edge of the tear. This has often been obscured by disturbance of the underlying cortex in your early attempts to locate and pick up the edge. In this case, use some trypan blue to enhance its visibility. You may want to retract the iris locally with a Kuglen hook (or similar) or dilate the pupil using iris microretractor hooks to obtain better exposure.

The first surgical option in this situation is one of the most valuable practical surgical tips that I know. It is your 'get out of jail free' card for retrieving a tear-out (Fig. 7.9). First, stop everything and ensure that the chamber is completely filled with viscoelastic. The secret is now to UNFOLD the flap and flatten it back on to its underlying bed of cortex. Then, using forceps, grasp the peripheral edge of the unfolded flap as near as practically possible

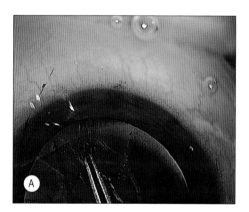
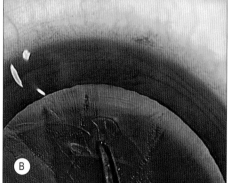
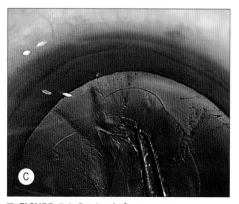
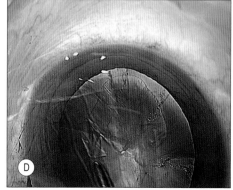

FIGURE 7.9 Retrieval of a tear-out.

behind the apex of the tear. Now pull on the flap directly backward circumferentially, making sure that the traction is applied in the plane of the capsule. Then, once it is under tension, pull it gently inward toward the center. This combination of traction applied backward and centrally to the unfolded flap resolves into a vector force that redirects the tear centrally. It does so at a much more acute angle than is possible if the free edge of the flap is left folded over and pulled forward and centrally in the 'normal' way.

If you are unlucky and the tear has extended far out into the zonules, then it will be irretrievable even with the above technique. Try it first, but if there is horizontal movement of the whole lens without any redirection of the tear in response to traction on the flap then you should release the flap, otherwise the tear may wrap around the equator and result in a dropped nucleus. How hard can you safely pull? The answer is, of course, just slightly less hard than you pulled the last time when the tear wrapped around the equator. Impossible to answer and learned only through experience but well worth practising in the wet lab using pig eyes, which are excellent for this purpose, or the more recently available high-grade model surgical eyes for CCC and phaco (Phillips Studio).

If you are faced with such an irretrievable tear-out, you have two remaining options. The first is to create a new starting point with capsule scissors by making a circumferential cut at a suitable radius in the leading edge of the tear and then continue around in the direction you were going (or use a can opener technique if you cannot manage this). The second is to complete the rhexis from the opposite direction (Fig. 7.10). In either case, you may be left with a discontinuous rhexis with a highly vulnerable peripheral tear-out. Prevention of further complications is your priority at this stage, and the available options for achieving this will depend on your confidence level, previous experience of such complications, available instrumentation, and surgical skills.

Extreme care is required. Do not try to be a hero. By definition, heroes take risks that are considered unacceptable by the majority of their peers, and remember that your peers are your judges. Always play safe and kick for touch. For most of us, this would involve cutting a relieving radial incision in the capsule diametrically opposite the tear-out (Fig. 7.11), and then carefully prolapsing the nucleus into the chamber using gentle hydrodissection or viscoelevation. Sandwich the nucleus between some dispersive viscoelastic in front to protect the endothelium and some behind to keep the capsular bag inflated, and then phaco the nucleus in the chamber (often referred to optimistically as supracapsular or iris plane).

You have to remind yourself at this stage that your primary interest is the best possible outcome for the patient. If

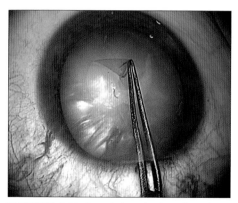

■ **FIGURE 7.10** Completion of a rhexis from the opposite direction.

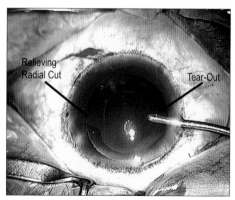

■ **FIGURE 7.11** A relieving radial incision in the capsule diametrically opposite the tear-out.

you are not confident to continue, then be brave enough to stop and close the eye. There is absolutely no shame in doing this, as it may well be the safest option. The operation can then be completed as soon as practically possible by a more experienced colleague, who you should assist. This way, you not only get to learn something but also the patient is more likely to get a good result.

Finally comes the choice of intraocular lens (IOL) to implant in such cases. Silicone plate haptic lenses are contraindicated because of their tendency to slip out of the bag through an incomplete rhexis. Some surgeons advocate the careful placement of a normal endocapsular IOL into the bag as usual, with the proviso that the haptics are oriented perpendicular to the diametrically oriented anterior capsule tear and relieving cut. Others prefer to select a sulcus-mounted posterior chamber lens (with suitable power reduction of 0.5 diopters). Sulcus implantation minimizes the risk of a wraparound tear with vitreous loss, which can still happen not only during endocapsular IOL implantation but also when removing viscoelastic from such a vulnerable capsular bag. Be aware that most IOLs that have been designed for endocapsular placement are NOT suitable for sulcus placement, as they are too small (≤ 12.5 mm), leading to instability and decentration, and/or have haptics that are too bulky and will chafe against the iris.

Summary

The two overwhelmingly important principles to take on board regarding radial tear-out of the capsulorrhexis are as follow.

1. Prevention is better than cure: stick to the basic principles for avoidance.
2. Stop at the very earliest sign of deviation of the rhexis, i.e. before you are in trouble.

Once it has undeniably happened, then the technique of unfolding the flap and pulling it circumferentially backward and then centrally is extraordinarily successful at retrieving the rhexis against seemingly impossible odds. If this does not work, then the choice between continuing with either endocapsular or anterior chamber phaco is that of individual surgeons and depends on their clinical judgment based on experience.

In principle, always take the safest route; this may be to call for help or, if none is on hand, to close the eye and let a more experienced surgeon complete the operation as soon as practically possible.

Some other general thoughts to reflect on are as follow.

- Practice does not make perfect—it just makes permanent.
- Proper preparation prevents poor performance.
- Trying very hard is the first step on the road to failure.

Good surgeons are those who have the insight to recognize when they are out of control, the humility to admit it, and the self-discipline to take effective action early on. They should also have the experience and adaptability to select, as well as the skill to calmly execute, the most appropriate and safest surgical exit strategy when faced with complications.

When you are older you tend to think about what can go wrong, while when you are younger you only think about what can go right.

REFERENCES

1. Neuhann T. [Theory and surgical technique of capsulorrhexis.] Klin Monatsbl Augenheilkol 1987; 190:542–545. (In German.)

2. Gimbel HV, Neuhann T. Continuous curvilinear capsulorrhexis. J Cataract Refract Surg 1991; 17:110–111.

FURTHER READING

Gimbel HV, Kaye GB. Forceps puncture continuous curvilinear capsulorrhexis. J Cataract Refract Surg 1997; 23:473–475.

Hausmann N, Richard G. Investigations on diathermy for anterior capsulotomy. Invest Ophthalmol Vis Sci 1991; 32:2155–2159.

Hoffer KJ, McFarland JE. Intracameral subcapsular fluorescein staining for improved visualisation during capsulorrhexis in mature cataracts. J Cataract Refract Surg 1993; 19:566.

Krag S, Thim K, Corydon L. Diathermic capsulotomy versus capsulorrhexis: a biomechanical study. J Cataract Refract Surg 1997; 23:86–90.

Melles GRJ, Waard PWT, Pameyer JH, et al. Trypan blue capsule staining to visualise the capsulorrhexis in cataract surgery. J Cataract Refract Surg 1999; 24:7–9.

Newsom TH, Oetting TN. Idocyanine green staining in traumatic cataract. J Cataract Refract Surg 2000; 26:1691–1693.

Nishi O, Nishi K, Wickstrom K. Preventing lens epithelial cell migration using intraocular lenses with sharp rectangular edges. J Cataract Refract Surg 2000; 26:1543–1549.

Teus MA, Fangundez-Vargas MA, Calvo MA, et al. Viscoelastic injecting cystotome. J Cataract Refract Surg 1998; 24:1432–1433.

8

Hydrodissection

Hydrodissection is the injection of balanced salt solution between the capsule and the peripheral soft lens matter. It is used to mobilize the nuclear–epinuclear complex within the capsular bag, and it is essential for all techniques of nucleus removal.

HYDRODELINEATION

This is the injection of fluid between the nucleus and the epinucleus, or soft lens matter, in order to separate the two components of the nuclear complex and to make some forms of nucleus removal easier.

HYDRODISSECTION

8.1

Figure 8.1 shows a 27-gauge hydrodissection cannula, which preferably is attached to a 2.5-mL syringe with a Luer-lok to stop it detaching because of the high pressures generated during hydrodissection. There are a number of designs for these cannulae; the one shown is round in cross-section and delivers a reasonable flow of fluid. Finer cannulae may produce a very high pressure jet and should probably be avoided. Some have a flattened cross-section, which is supposed to make the passage of fluid between the capsule and the peripheral cortex spread out more easily. The cannula shown in Figure 8.1 is a Bolger-type cannula designed for a technique called cortical cleavage hydrodissection.[1] Howard Fine described this technique, involving a very peripheral injection, to cleave the anterior capsule from the peripheral cortex. The main advantage of this technique is that there is very little soft lens matter remaining after

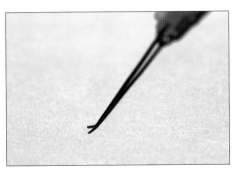

FIGURE 8.1 A Bolger-style hydrodissection cannula with a relatively large tip to obtain good flow of balanced salt solution during hydrodissection. The tip is rounded and safe for use in the capsular bag.

nucleus removal, and very little need for irrigation–aspiration or cortical cleanup.

Figure 8.2 shows a simple technique to ensure peripheral placement of the hydrodissection cannula. The cannula is inserted into the anterior chamber, which is still full of viscoelastic from the capsulorrhexis. The tip of the cannula is laid on top of the anterior capsule, and is then moved gently backward until it just slips under the edge of the rhexis, whence injection can begin and a fluid wave is propagated in the very peripheral cortical region. Steady pressure should be maintained to ensure that the fluid wave passes backward around the periphery of the lens, and a fluid wave should be observed moving across the entire dimension of the lens. If this is not observed, injection in another site should be tried until a definite fluid wave had been seen.

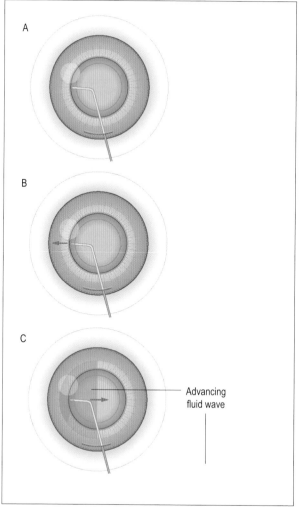

A

B

C

Advancing
fluid wave

■ **FIGURE 8.2 (A)** The cannula resting on top of the anterior capsulorrhexis edge. **(B)** It is gently moved centrally until it just falls off the edge of the rhexis and on to the surface of the cortical lens matter, when injection can begin. **(C)** It is advanced peripherally again, and injection pressure is maintained as the advancing fluid wave is seen spreading across the back surface of the lens.

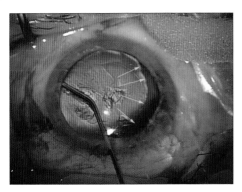

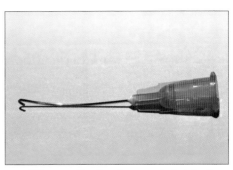

■ **FIGURE 8.4** The Corydon cannula for injecting fluid around the subincisional cortex.

■ **FIGURE 8.3** The advancing fluid wave, with the edge outlined by arrows.

Figure 8.3 shows a fluid wave moving across the posterior aspect of the lens. As the fluid wave moves around the back of the lens and starts to dissect the lens fibers opposite to the site of injection, continued pressure will sometimes cause expression of the nuclear complex out of the capsular bag. The hydrodissection cannula can be used to gently replace the nucleus if it is moving forward. Some surgeons prefer multiple injection sites to ensure that all the peripheral cortical matter is freed up, but this is generally unnecessary if a good fluid wave has been observed. The hydrodissection cannula tip should be kept at 90° to the rhexis edge if possible at all times, to ensure an even spread of fluid, but if multiple injection sites are used, this rule can be broken, as fluid will be injected from different directions. Occasionally, if zonular stress is to be avoided, for example in a case of advanced pseudoexfoliation, then a technique called viscoexpression can be used.

Figure 8.4 shows a Corydon U-shaped cannula, which can be used with viscoelastic to inject under the capsule at the subincisional position; this will often gently elevate the nucleus out of the bag, with very little zonular stress. This same cannula can be used with balanced salt solution if the subincisional area is difficult to free with routine hydrodissection.

CAPSULAR BLOCK SYNDROME

This occurs when forcible hydrodissection is performed in an eye with a hard nucleus and a small capsulorrhexis. As the fluid wave passes around the back of the lens, the nucleus is pushed forward and effectively closes off the capsulorrhexis opening. Further rapid injection of fluid from the hydrodissection cannula can result in rapid distension of the capsular bag. If this goes unnoticed, even further injection will rupture the posterior capsule, at which time a phenomenon called pupil snap occurs, when the whole iris lens diaphragm suddenly snaps backward. Even this event may go unobserved, and if phacoemulsification is attempted, inevitably the nucleus will tumble into the vitreous cavity, as there is no posterior support.

To prevent this phenomenon, if an eye has a hard nucleus and a small rhexis, then, as injection is occurring, the hydrodissection cannula should be used to gently 'ballot' the nucleus backward, thus forcing fluid back up into the anterior chamber and preventing the build-up of fluid between the nucleus and posterior capsule.

HYDRODELINEATION

This is a useful technique to outline the size of the nucleus during a chopping technique, and also limit the size of the material to be removed by phacoemulsification, thereby also limiting the energy put into the eye. In addition, the epinucleus, which is left behind, is protective for the posterior capsule but clearly needs to be removed by irrigation–aspiration at the end of the phaco maneuver. For this technique, the same hydrodissection cannula is used, after an initial hydrodissection. Hydrodelineation involves placing the cannula into the soft lens matter, in the midperiphery, and injecting fluid between the lens nucleus and the epinucleus. As the fluid wave passes around the edge of the nucleus, the edge is clearly delineated and can be seen as a so-called golden ring sign (Figs 8.5 and 8.6).

Successful hydrodissection and/or hydrodelineation should result in a freely mobile nucleus or nuclear–cortical complex. Failure to achieve this should encourage further hydro-dissection until it does occur.

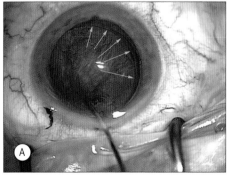 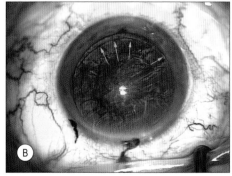

■ **FIGURE 8.5** (**A**) The golden ring (arrows) is the delineation between the harder central nucleus and the softer cortical matter. (**B**) The golden ring is seen better once the injection is complete (arrows).

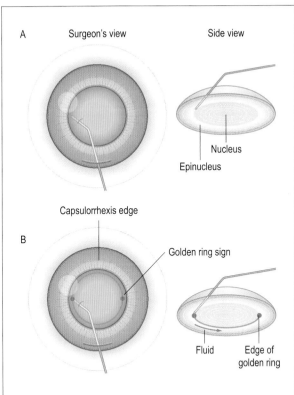

A — Surgeon's view — Side view

Nucleus
Epinucleus

Capsulorrhexis edge

B

Golden ring sign

Fluid — Edge of golden ring

■ **FIGURE 8.6** Hydrodelineation: the golden ring sign. (**A**) The hydrodelineation cannula is plunged into the soft lens matter until resistance is felt. (**B**) Fluid is forced between the soft lens matter and the nucleus, creating a fluid interface that is seen as the golden ring.

REFERENCE

1. Fine IH. Cortical cleavage hydrodissection. J Cataract Refract Surg 1992; 18:508–512.

9

Nuclear strategies

INSTRUMENTATION

Coaxial instruments are:

- the phacoemulsification probe;
- the second instrument;
- viscoelastic; and
- microgrooved or colibri forceps.

Bimanual instruments are:

- a bimanual unsleeved phaco probe;
- an irrigating chopper; and
- microcapsulorrhexis forceps.

Flexibility in the surgical approach to nucleus removal is essential. It is therefore necessary to learn a number of different techniques, which will allow free conversion from one to the other during a case and between cases. The surgeon may choose to have one favorite technique, but the ability to switch to other techniques is essential in order to cope with the range of cataracts presenting, and indeed the intraoperative complications that may occur. Essentially, there are three main types of technique that are useful for dealing with soft, medium, and hard cataract. Generically, they can be called chip and flip, divide and conquer, and chopping techniques, respectively.

A slit-lamp assessment of the cataract concerned will reveal details of its nature and possibly its hardness. The patient's age will influence the degree of nuclear sclerosis, and trauma may play a part in the type of cataract formed. The patient's corneal endothelium must be assessed, as a poorly functioning endothelium may demand a shorter operation, with less fluid flow through the eye, less energy in the eye, and possibly a scleral tunnel approach. Nuclear white scatter cataract can produce a greater refractive change than nuclear sclerosis, and in my experience these types of cataract are much harder than nuclear sclerotic cataract. Nuclear white scatter cataracts have a milky appearance and can be a little more difficult to assess, because they sometimes cause more subtle optical changes in the nucleus than a nuclear sclerotic cataract does. Once the hardness of the nucleus has been assessed, the type of procedure for nucleus removal can be selected, and this may influence the equipment needed and set up by the theater team.

SOFT CATARACTS
Chip and flip

9.1

Children and young adults often have soft lenses, and sometimes no phacoemulsification is required at all, as the lens is soft enough to aspirate. I still use a phaco probe for these cases, as it provides a very good instrument for aspiration, and just occasionally there is a little nuclear hardness that needs to be dealt with, especially in trauma cases.

Chip and flip involves making a deep central groove, almost the diameter of the lens (the "chip"), and demands excellent hydrodissection. Even despite this, some of these younger nuclei can be very difficult to rotate because of their gelatinous nature, and it is sometimes easier to simply aspirate various parts of the lens, and manipulate other parts into position for removal, and there can sometimes be very little structure to the process. However, with some slight firmness of the nucleus, a deep central groove is made and the nucleus rotated through 180° to complete the full-length groove. This should be as deep as possible. The phaco probe and second instrument are then used to separate the two halves, as far as possible, and for these cases a paddlelike second instrument is very useful, as it has a greater surface area. Once the two halves have been separated, one half is rotated into position, opposite the phaco tip, and the tip gently embedded in the lens matter. High vacuum is then used to aspirate the nucleus out of the capsular bag (the flip); although sometimes phacoemulsification is required, it is more often a phaco-assisted aspiration used to remove the soft lens. The second half is then rotated opposite the phaco probe and the process repeated.

The procedure can be very quick indeed with a very soft cataract, and care must be taken, if very high vacuums are being generated, that a postocclusion surge does not occur. However, because of the soft nature of the cataract, this is less likely, as total blockage does not usually occur (see next section for details of postocclusion surge). Figure 9.1 shows the various stages of the chip and flip procedure.

MEDIUM CATARACTS
Divide and conquer

9.2

This is a good default technique taught to most beginning cataract surgeons, and can also be used as a fallback procedure if another nuclear strategy is not progressing satisfactorily. Its use aims to divide the nucleus into four roughly equal parts, and then use high vacuum and phaco energy to remove ('conquer') them. Phacoemulsification should take place in the safe central part of the anterior chamber, within the vertical constraints of the capsular bag, to make it as safe as possible.

Beginning surgeons should choose nuclei between grade 2 and 3, as anything softer would be difficult to crack, or

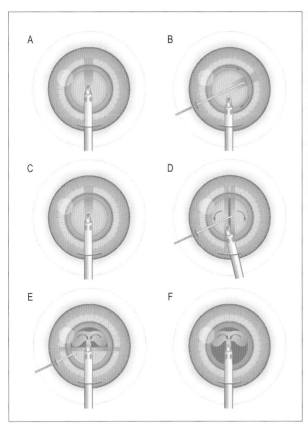

■ **FIGURE 9.1** The stages of a chip and flip technique. (**A**) A deep central groove is made. (**B**) The nucleus is rotated 180°. (**C**) The groove is completed to be almost the diameter of the lens. (**D**) The nucleus is split into two. This step can be difficult, as the nucleus is often soft and gelatinous. (**E**) The heminuclei are rotated so that they are opposite the phaco probe. (**F**) Using high vacuum, the soft nucleus is flipped out of the capsular bag and into the phaco probe, using phaco-assisted aspiration. The second heminucleus is then rotated and the process repeated.

divide, and anything harder will take a long time and generate a lot of energy in the eye.

Initial sculpting

The phaco probe is put into the eye with continuous irrigation on, or the foot switch in position 1, to ensure that fluid maintains the anterior chamber depth at all times. The bevel of the phaco probe can be inserted facing downward, but then needs to be rotated to face upward once it is in the eye. Care must be taken not to snag Descemet's membrane as the probe is put into the eye, as this can be stripped from the inner aspect of the cornea quite easily, resulting in corneal decompensation. It is important to remember the valve-like effect that the wound has due to its shape, and also to enter the eye in a relatively downward position, rather than trying to push the probe into the stroma.

Once inside the eye, position 1 on the foot pedal is maintained, and the second instrument can be placed into the anterior chamber through the side port. Position 2 is reached with the foot pedal, and the pump in the peristaltic machine will start to turn, generating aspiration. As fluid is sucked out of the eye, it is replaced, by gravity, from the bottle above the machine. At this point, it is worth noting that there is chamber stability before depressing the pedal into position 3 to start the phaco tip vibrating. This must be done before the needle is moved against the cataract. A common mistake with beginning phaco surgeons is to try to push the phaco needle against the cataract before foot position 3 has been reached. This simply causes stress on superior zonules and will move the whole capsular–nuclear complex away from the surgeon. If this movement is seen to occur, then successive sculpts should be shallower, slower, or both to allow easy passage of the needle through the cataractous material, with no movement of the nucleus. The eye itself may be seen to move, but the nucleus and bag should remain stationary as the probe traverses across the nuclear surface and removes material. There can be a slight tendency to gouge the cataract; this should be avoided.

As successive sculpts are made, the groove is widened to allow passage of the irrigating sleeve, as well as the phaco needle. Once the needle is below the depth of the capsulorrhexis, longer passes can be made, remembering to move the needle upward at the end of the groove, as the cataract is thinner peripherally and capsule damage can occur if the trench is made all one depth.

A good guide to depth within the nucleus is the appearance of the posterior Y suture (see Fig. 9.2). Once the phaco needle has passed through this plane, the nucleus will be much easier to disassemble. The nucleus is then rotated through 90° with the second instrument, which is impaled deeply into the wall of the trench, furthest from the hand in which the second instrument is held. A deliberate, purposeful rotation of the second instrument between finger and thumb is then made, using the bend in the instrument as a fulcrum. This rotatory movement is uniplanar and will result in the breakdown of any residual lens capsule adhesions. Sometimes, the hydrodissection is incomplete and initial resistance is felt, but if sustained pressure is maintained on the rotating instrument, the nucleus will eventually give way and start to rotate slowly. The sculpting is

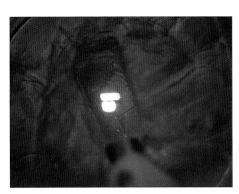

■ **FIGURE 9.2** A high-magnification image showing the posterior Y suture (arrows). This is a good landmark, because, once this has been passed, the depth of the groove is about two-thirds of the lens thickness.

then repeated at 90° to the initial trench the same way, and the process repeated until four mutually perpendicular trenches have been cut (Fig. 9.3).

At this point, it is worth taking a moment just to assess the depth of the grooves. If the peripheral posterior cortical lens matter has been reached, a feathery or silvery appearance in the base of the trench will be seen. Another guide that sufficient depth has been reached is that the trench should be two to three times as deep as the diameter of the phaco needle, which is about 1 mm. Once sufficient depth has been created, the nucleus can be cracked. This is most easily achieved if the phaco probe is positioned deep in the groove, opposite the phaco wound, and held still. The second

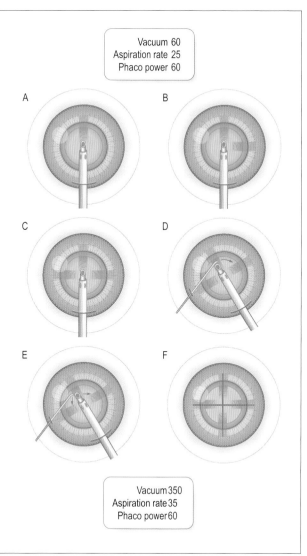

■ **FIGURE 9.3** The divide and conquer technique. (**A**) An initial groove is made by sculpting. (**B**) The nucleus is rotated, and a second groove is made at 90° to the first. (**C**) This is repeated until four grooves mutually at right angles exist. (**D**) Cross action splitting. The phaco probe is placed deep in the base of one of the grooves and used as a stopper. The second instrument is pushed away from the phaco probe to commence nuclear fracture. (**E**) Uncrossed splitting. Alternatively, the two instruments can be moved apart in the opposite direction. (**F**) The nucleus is rotated and the nuclear fracture repeated in all four quadrants. All four quadrants split.

instrument can then be used to push against the right-hand wall of the trench (for right-handed surgeons), using the phaco probe as a stop against which to push (Fig. 9.4). A crack will be seen to propagate through the posterior lens plate and along most of its length. If this does not occur, the instruments are either too shallow in the trench or the trench itself is not deep enough. Once a crack has occurred, the nucleus is rotated through 90° and the process repeated. This is done in all four trenches.

Once the nucleus is divided in this way, the settings on the phacoemulsification machine are changed to give a high preset vacuum and a faster aspiration rate, and either pulsed or burst mode for the phaco mode are favored by some surgeons. This ensures that, as pieces are attracted to the phaco tip by vacuum (sucking) and flow induced by aspiration (pushing), they are less likely to be repelled by the force of the phaco needle vibrating. The divided nucleus is positioned so that one quadrant is opposite the phaco tip. The tip of the needle is occluded against the nucleus, and position 2 of the foot pedal is maintained. This allows vacuum to build up to the preset level; once this happens, a warning sound will be heard. The nuclear fragment can then be lifted into the safe central zone, position 3 engaged, and the fragment emulsified (Fig. 9.5). If the cataract is very brittle or hard, using a second instrument to tip up the quadrant being removed can be a useful maneuver to avoid the sharp lower edges coming into contact with the posterior capsule as the fragment is emulsified (Fig. 9.6). As the last quadrant is removed, the second instrument can be placed below the nuclear fragment to ensure that, if a postocclusion surge occurs, the posterior capsule is not damaged by coming into contact with the vibrating needle (Fig. 9.7). This can be anticipated by allowing the foot pedal into position 1 just before the last fragment is seen to disappear into the phaco tip.

9.4

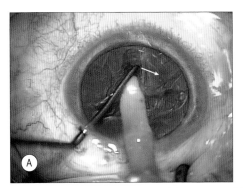
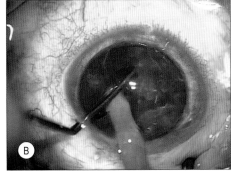

■ **FIGURE 9.4** (**A**) Clinical picture of the position of the instruments just before the first nuclear fracture is made. (**B**) The position of the instruments at the point of nucleus fracture.

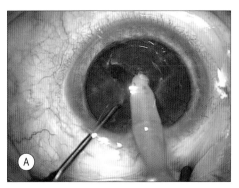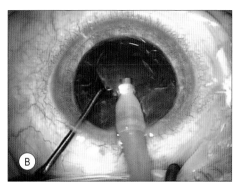

■ **FIGURE 9.5** (**A**) The first fragment is lifted into the safe central zone for phacoemulsification using high vacuum. (**B**) The nucleus is rotated and a second fragment lifted into the center.

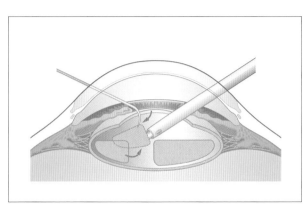

■ **FIGURE 9.6** Tipping the nuclear fragment. The technique is used to elevate the first fragment if it is locked between other fragments, to avoid a sharp posterior aspect of the nucleus impinging on the capsule as aspiration is attempted.

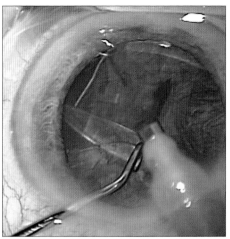

■ **FIGURE 9.7** During removal of the last fragment, the second instrument (in this case a chopper) is held underneath the tip of the phaco probe to prevent posterior capsule damage if post-occlusion surge occurs.

Post-occlusion surge

A number of modern machines have inbuilt mechanisms to try to prevent postocclusion surge, including an array of sensors and pump controls, which are designed to keep the anterior chamber formed at all times. A postocclusion surge usually occurs when a high vacuum has been obtained during phacoemulsification of a fragment, and the fragment has occluded the tip of the phaco probe, allowing the vacuum to build up. As the fragment is emulsified, flow begins once again very rapidly up the needle once the blockage has been removed. As the vacuum is at a very high preset level, this sudden surge of fluid into the needle can collapse the chamber, because fluid is not being replaced quickly enough from the irrigating bottle.

Alcon (Fort Worth, Texas) have overcome this by using a so-called aspiration bypass system. This comprises a small hole in the side of the phaco tip, which allows some flow of fluid back up the needle even if the tip is occluded, and means that flow is maintained at all times. This is especially important for cooling the needle, but also means that there is not such a big pressure drop once the fragment has been emulsified. Non-compliant tubing is another mechanism used to avoid postocclusion surge, but awareness of its existence and anticipation of its occurrence can be useful ways of avoiding it.

HARD CATARACTS

Chopping techniques

9.5

Phaco chop was originally described by Nagahara.[1] Chopping techniques can be broadly divided into those that utilize a deep central groove and those that do not. Nagahara described the latter, which is perhaps a little more difficult to learn but may be slightly quicker.

Phaco chop (horizontal chopping)

Figure 9.8 outlines the steps in the phaco chop procedure. In this technique, excellent hydrodissection is required to ensure free nuclear rotation. The parameters for this are slightly different to those for standard phaco. It is important to have at least 3 mm of phaco tip protruding from the irrigating sleeve (assuming that coaxial phaco is being used). The phaco tip is introduced into the eye with the bevel down and the tip embedded into the central nucleus, using high vacuum and a little phaco power. The chopper is introduced under the edge of the capsulorrhexis and over the edge of the nucleus, and drawn toward the phaco tip and moved sideways just before they meet (Fig. 9.9). The phaco probe and chopper are angled away from each other in order to produce the first split in the nuclear complex; this process is repeated after the nucleus is rotated to produce a second fracture. The nuclear segments thus produced

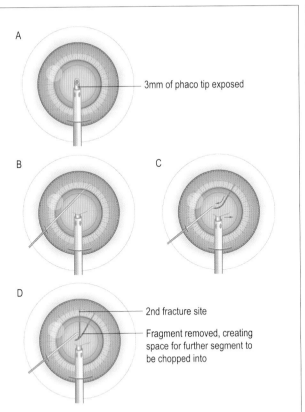

■ **FIGURE 9.8** The horizontal chop technique. (**A**) The phaco probe, with 3 mm of tip protruding from the irrigating sleeve, is driven into the nucleus, starting peripherally and ending up with the tip central in the nucleus. It is important to ensure that the irrigation holes are in the anterior chamber to maintain the chamber depth and flow of fluid. (**B**) The chopper is manipulated into position, under the capsulorrhexis edge and over the edge of the nucleus. (**C**) The chopper is drawn toward the tip of the phaco probe and at the last moment swept aside to create a nucleus fracture. (**D**) The nucleus is rotated and the process repeated, causing a fragment to fracture off the main body of the nucleus. This can then be aspirated and emulsified.

A — 3mm of phaco tip exposed

B

C

D — 2nd fracture site

Fragment removed, creating space for further segment to be chopped into

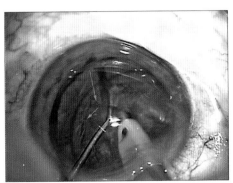

■ **FIGURE 9.9** Clinical picture showing the direction of movement of the chopper, initially toward the phaco probe and then away from it to create the nucleus fracture.

are aspirated into the central area of the anterior chamber and emulsified. The remaining nucleus is rotated, and the process repeated until all fragments are removed. Some surgeons prefer to position the chopper over the edge of the nucleus before impaling the phaco probe into the central nucleus. This provides some stability while the phaco tip is embedded into the nucleus.

Stop and chop

Originally described by Paul Koch,[2] this technique is a little easier to learn, as it involves the familiar sculpting technique and provides a space into which to chop nuclear fragments. The name derives from the fact that the central sculpting is stopped after a groove the diameter of the lens is made; the procedure then converts to a chop technique.

9.6

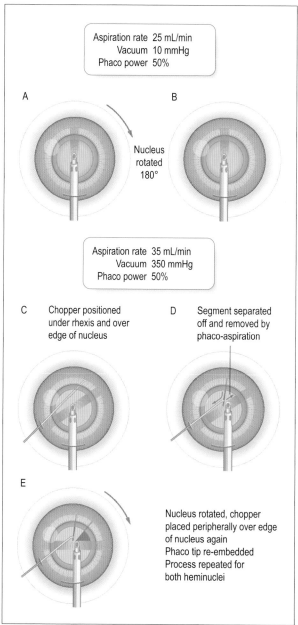

Aspiration rate 25 mL/min
Vacuum 10 mmHg
Phaco power 50%

A

B

Nucleus
rotated
180°

Aspiration rate 35 mL/min
Vacuum 350 mmHg
Phaco power 50%

C   Chopper positioned
under rhexis and over
edge of nucleus

D   Segment separated
off and removed by
phaco-aspiration

E

Nucleus rotated, chopper
placed peripherally over edge
of nucleus again
Phaco tip re-embedded
Process repeated for
both heminuclei

■ **FIGURE 9.10** The stop and chop technique. (**A**) A groove is made in the usual way. (**B**) The nucleus is rotated and the groove completed to be virtually the diameter of the lens. (**C**) The nucleus is rotated about 30° and the tip of the phaco probe impaled into the nucleus using high vacuum. The chopper is positioned under the rhexis and over the edge of the nucleus. (**D**) The chopper is drawn toward the tip of the phaco probe and moved sideways at the last moment to create a nucleus fracture. (**E**) Because of the existence of the central groove, there is room to easily remove this chopped fragment. The nucleus is then rotated and the process repeated for both heminuclei.

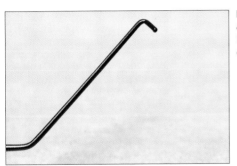

■ **FIGURE 9.11** A close up of a chopper (Duckworth & Kent). The inner aspect of the terminal part of the instrument is sharp, but the very end is blunt to ensure that it is capsule-friendly.

Figure 9.10 shows the stop and chop technique in its various stages. Having completed the deep central groove, almost the diameter of the lens, the nucleus is turned through 30° and the tip of the phaco probe embedded with high vacuum into the wall of the nuclear trench. A chopping instrument (Fig. 9.11) is introduced through the side port, carefully placed under the edge of the capsulorrhexis, and positioned at the edge of the nucleus. The chopper is then drawn toward the phaco tip and, just before they meet, swept sideways to separate the nuclear fragment. The fragment can then be removed by aspiration and phacoemulsification. Again, some surgeons prefer pulse or burst mode at this point. The nucleus is then further rotated and the procedure repeated until the whole heminucleus has been removed. The second heminucleus is then rotated into position and the procedure repeated until all fragments are removed.

Vertical chopping

Vertical chopping is useful for very hard nuclei and has the advantage that the chopper is kept within the capsulorrhexis area. It is a little more difficult to master, but entails the impaled phaco probe in the central nucleus being lifted as the vertical chopper is depressed in the opposite direction, causing a vertical fracture to occur through the nucleus (see Fig. 9.12). The fragments are removed and further fracture lines produced in the same way. This technique has some merit in terms of safety, in that the chopping action is started within the confines of the capsulorrhexis margin, and the chopper does not have to be placed peripherally over the edge of the nucleus. However, the action of vertical chop is a little more difficult to get used to and is not a good technique to learn phaco chopping with.

Laser phacoemulsification

Yttrium–aluminum–garnet (YAG) lasers have been available for a number of years. The two main mechanisms used are the Dodick (neodymium:YAG) laser,[3] which relies on laser energy being converted to mechanical energy at the tip of a probe by vibrating a titanium plate, and the Wavelight

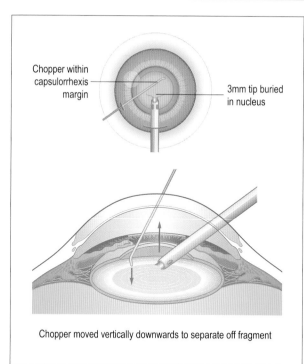

Chopper within capsulorrhexis margin

3mm tip buried in nucleus

Chopper moved vertically downwards to separate off fragment

■ **FIGURE 9.12** The vertical chop technique. The phaco probe is driven deep into the center of the nucleus, again starting peripherally and ending up centrally, and ensuring that the irrigating holes are within the anterior chamber. The chopper is placed much more centrally and, as the two instruments are drawn toward each other, the nucleus is lifted upward, via the phaco probe, and the chopper depressed downward, to create a vertical fracture. Specialized choppers can be used but even a Sinskey hook can work.

erbium:YAG, which depends on a coupling effect of hydroxyl ions in water and the laser energy at 2.94 μm. Because of the high absorption coefficient in water, cavitation with bubble formation occurs in the eye, which has a disruptive effect, the penetration depth of which is 0.1 mm in water and 0.05 mm in tissue (the lens).[4] The main advantages of these systems is that there is minimal heat generated, and the risk of phaco burns is virtually zero. In my experience with the Wavelight laser, it is useful for soft cataracts but is slow when used for moderate to hard cataracts. The feel of the surgery is somewhat different, as the tip of the phaco probe does not vibrate at all but lens disruption is caused by the cavitation effect of the laser being delivered from the resonance chamber of the laser machine down a zirconium fluoride fiber with a quartz tip. Thus the effect of lens disruption is visible but not palpable. Another advantage of the erbium:YAG laser is that probes for capsulorrhexis and vitrectomy are also available, and the one machine can drive all three probes. This might make such a machine suitable for pediatric cataracts, which are very soft, and in which an anterior and posterior capsulorrhexis are often required.

The Dodick laser has been used extensively in the USA, and large prospective studies have been published.[5] A variety of methods can be used to remove the nucleus with these lasers; either divide and conquer or phaco chop are popular.

OTHER METHODS OF CATARACT REMOVAL

Phacoemulsification has been adopted in many developed countries, but remains expensive in terms of both capital expenditure and equipment maintenance. Other methods of cataract removal include intracapsular and extracapsular techniques, as well as small incision, sutureless, non-phaco surgery. Lensectomy is another technique used especially in pediatric cases, where phacoemulsification may not be necessary due to the softness of the cataract. These will be described in turn.

Intracapsular cataract extraction

There are rarely indications for this nowadays, but it was a popular technique in the 1950s through to the 1970s. Nowadays, if phacoemulsification or extracapsular surgery cannot be completed safely, for example in a grossly dislocated lens, it may be safer to carry out a pars planar lensectomy rather than attempt an intracapsular extraction and risk vitreous loss and vitreoretinal traction.

The technique involved making a large (140°) scleral or corneal incision, the exact size of which could be guided by the expected size of the lens being extracted, a very elderly cataract needing a greater cord length to be pulled out of the eye than a younger one. Often, preplaced sutures were used in the cornea or sclera, which were swept aside as the cornea was manipulated forward and the wound opened. The iris was then retracted out of the way, often with a dry sponge, and a cryoprobe touched on to the lens capsule and its pedal depressed to initiate a freeze. As soon as an ice ball was seen to form through the lens capsule and into the lens substance, gentle manipulations of the lens were made side to side to break any residual zonular fibers (zonulysin or alphachymotripsin was used to dissolve the zonules first). The lens was then gently lifted out of the eye, allowing a short period of time to elapse before the lens was fully removed from the eye, to allow any vitreous adhesions to break. Once the lens was removed, the anterior chamber was re-formed with balanced salt solution (often Hartmann's solution in those days) and an implant inserted into the eye, if one was available.

Anterior chamber lenses were popular, as were iris clip lenses, and a number of the older-style lenses gave significant problems, the history of which is outlined magnificently in a DVD manufactured for the Moorfields Eye Hospital, London, bicentenary celebrations, and written and presented by Hugh Williams, called *Casanova and the Spitfire Pilots*.

It was not uncommon for the lens capsule to rupture as it was pulled out of the eye, or for vitreous to accompany the lens as it was removed. Aphakic glaucoma was another complication that often arose, probably because with scleral wounds a large contingent of the trabecular meshwork

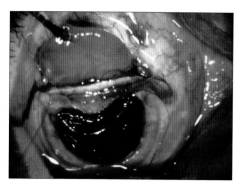

■ **FIGURE 9.13** A lens being extracted by intracapsular technique. Note the severe folding of the cornea as the lens is removed.

TABLE 9.1 Comparison of corneal and scleral section

Section	Advantages	Disadvantages
Corneal	Quicker No bleeding 'Mechanics easier' (more stable) No superior rectus suture needed Easier access for trabeculectomy later	More astigmatism Endothelial damage Suture care (loose etc.) Less strong wound
Scleral	Less astigmatism Wound alignment easier Less endothelial damage Suture care less (below conjunctiva) Stronger wound	More bleeding Astigmatism less easily changed (by removing sutures) More trabecular meshwork damage Postoperative intraocular pressure rise more likely Iris prolapse more likely May need superior rectus suture Trabeculectomy more difficult later Takes longer

was initially cut and subsequently fibrosed postoperatively. Figure 9.13 shows an intracapsular cataract extraction at the time of nucleus removal.

Extracapsular cataract extraction

This can be done by either a corneal or a scleral wound, the pros and cons of which are shown in Table 9.1.

9.7

Corneal wound

This should be made with a predictably and consistently sharp knife. A diamond-bladed knife is perfect for the job, as it retains its sharp edge for many cases. The corneal wound should be made either perpendicular to the surface of the eye or slightly backward-sloping with respect to the corneal surface. This makes it self-sealing and much easier to accurately appose the edges. The size of the wound, and the length therefore of the cord through which the nucleus must be expressed, depends on the size and hardness of the nucleus, which must be judged at the slit lamp preopera-

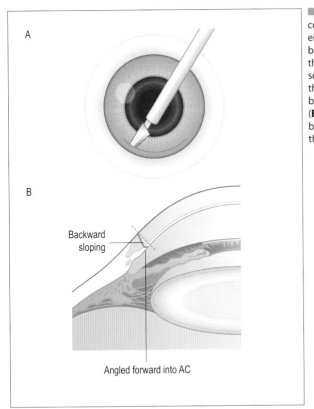

A

B

Backward
sloping

Angled forward into AC

■ **FIGURE 9.14** Construction of a corneal wound. The wound is made either perpendicular or slightly backward-sloping (**A**) with respect to the corneal surface to ensure that it is self-sealing. The job of the sutures is then not to keep the wound closed, but simply to stop it opening. (**B**) The wound in cross-section, backward-sloping with respect to the surface of the cornea.

tively. The wound is backward-sloping for as deep as possible before entering the anterior chamber (see Fig. 9.14).

Scleral wound
The conjunctiva is reflected off the limbus, and the limbal wound is begun perpendicular to the surface of the eye for as deep as possible before dissecting forward between the scleral lamellae and into the clear cornea, at which point the anterior chamber is entered. This is a stepped wound, which is important because of the proximity of the wound to the iris root, which makes the likelihood of iris prolapse much greater if the wound is simply forward-sloping.

Capsulotomy
Traditionally, a so-called can-opener capsulotomy was utilized (see Fig. 9.15), and multiple perforations in the anterior capsule were made with a bent 27-gauge cystotome, which could be made by the surgeon by bending a needle or by using a preformed cystotome purchased commercially. It is also possible to perform a capsulorrhexis for this technique, but it is sensible to perform the capsulorrhexis through a small side-port incision before opening the main wound, in order to maintain the anterior chamber. The capsulotomy must be made large enough to express the

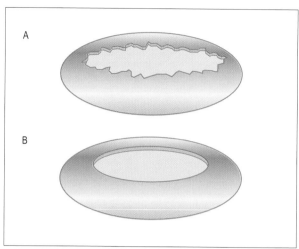

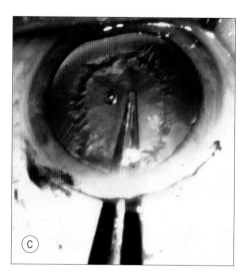

FIGURE 9.15 The difference between a ragged can-opener capsulotomy (**A**) and a smooth-edged capsulorrhexis (**B**). A can-opener capsulotomy about to be torn (**C**). Many microtears exist once the central portion has been removed; these are potential areas for capsular tearing during either nucleus expression or phacoemulsification.

nucleus, and therefore some idea of its size must be ascertained before this step. Hydrodissection is performed to loosen the nuclear complex, and then a blunt instrument is placed at the inferior limbus and pressure applied to the globe. Vitreous counterpressure forces the nucleus upward and out of the capsular bag, and gentle pressure on the anterior lip of the scleral or corneal wound opens the eye and allows the nucleus to slide out. If undue pressure is necessary, it is important to stop, re-form the anterior chamber, and make the wound larger in order not to rupture the posterior capsule during nucleus expression.

Once the nucleus has been expressed, the anterior chamber is often collapsed and needs to be re-formed rapidly with balanced salt solution. Irrigation aspiration of the soft lens matter is carried out with an instrument such as the Simcoe cannula, and a non-folding implant can be inserted under viscoelastic before the wound is sutured with either a continuous 'bootlace' type of suture or interrupted radial 10/0 nylon sutures. The continuous suture is perhaps quicker, and is supposed to give more even tension throughout its length. However, the main disadvantage of this type of suture is that, if it snaps anywhere along its length, it must be removed completely and the wound resutured if healing has not occurred yet. With interrupted sutures, they can be removed individually to help deal with residual astigmatism. Either way, care of the sutures is most important because, if they are left in situ for a year or longer, they will often snap or work loose. Patients should be warned that they may experience a foreign body feeling in the eye, and they should attend for suture removal if this is the case.

9.8

It is common that these sutures are overtightened and produce a steepening of the vertical meridian of the cornea. This would be corrected optically with a negative cylinder, with its axis at 180°. If this type of prescription is obtained following surgery, then it is often useful to remove the sutures 3 or 4 months after the operation, when a more spherical cornea can be anticipated, as the cornea flattens slightly in the vertical meridian with suture removal.

Poor suturing technique can cause side to side misalignment as well as steepening of the relevant meridian, and this can be a cause of dramatic postoperative visual disturbance. For this reason alone, the conversion to phacoemulsification can convert an average surgeon into a good one by taking away the necessity for extremely accurate wound alignment and suture technique. The technique of extracapsular surgery remains widespread throughout developing countries and can produce very good results, but close attention must be paid to the wound construction and suturing techniques.

Non-phaco, small-incision, sutureless cataract surgery

This is becoming popular in developing countries, as it provides a slightly smaller wound than an extracapsular operation, does not require suturing, and is quicker than the extracapsular technique with suturing. However, there are as yet no long-term data on endothelial survival and postoperative glaucoma rates, and the various methods of performing this type of surgery need careful evaluation if it is to become widespread. It is, however, a much cheaper form of surgery than phacoemulsification, and is likely to become very popular in the near future. Figure 9.16 shows the principles of this small-incision sutureless surgery. Basically, it is a scleral extracapsular wound that is constructed 2 mm from the limbus, with an initial perpendicular groove and a tunnel forward into the clear cornea. An angled entry into the anterior chamber is then made to form a stepped wound, and the extracapsular technique is aided by hydrodelineation, which ensures separation of the

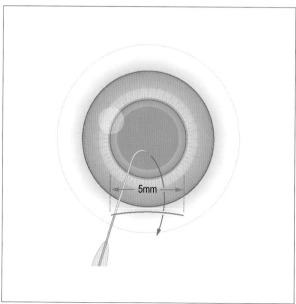

5mm

FIGURE 9.16 Sutureless, small-incision, extracapsular cataract extraction. A backward-sloping scleral tunnel is constructed, and good hydrodissection and hydrodelineation are performed to loosen the nucleus. A sharp instrument, such as a bent needle, can be used to engage the nucleus and deliver it out of the capsular bag. The incision can then be enlarged to 6 or 7 mm to insert an implant, and is usually stable enough to require no sutures. Here, the thoroughly hydrodissected and hydrodelineated nucleus is freely rotating.

harder nucleus. This can then be manipulated out of the eye with a sharp instrument, such as a modified cystotome, used as a fishhook. Irrigation–aspiration is carried out as for an extracapsular technique, and the wound can be enlarged to 6.5 or 7 mm for implantation of a non-folding implant. The wound is self-sealing because of its stepped nature, and reasonably strong.

PEDIATRIC CATARACT

Soft pediatric cataracts can often be removed with aspiration alone, but it is useful to use the phaco probe to start the process, because, by creating a central groove in the soft lens, it is much easier to subsequently aspirate the residual lens matter. The chip and flip method can be attempted, but sometimes the cataract is so soft that this can be difficult, and the lens matter is removed by a combination of aspiration and manipulations with a second instrument. Having completed the removal of the lens matter in children under the age of 10, it is useful to carry out a primary posterior capsulorrhexis and anterior vitrectomy. The intraocular lens implant, if used, can be placed with its haptics in the remaining peripheral capsular bag and the lens effectively buttonholed through the posterior capsulorrhexis.

Microincision cataract surgery

Microincision cataract surgery has become popular recently, as it allows smaller wounds to be used by separating the infusion and aspiration or phaco. Incisions as small as 1.5 mm can be used for microincision surgery, but new instrumentation has had to be developed. For example,

9.9

microcapsulorrhexis forceps, small enough to go through these wounds, are now available, as are a range of irrigating choppers, which, because of their small diameter, need to have a very high infusion bottle to maintain adequate inflow to the eye during surgery. This has all been made possible by the advent of energy modulation during pulse and burst modes, such as is provided in the White Star module from Allergan. This means that less heat is generated by the phaco needle, and it therefore does not need a cooling irrigation sleeve around it.

Because the irrigating chopper is a rigid instrument, it is difficult to seal the wound around this instrument; therefore leakage is quite a problem with this technique. That is another reason why a very high infusion bottle is needed to adequately replace the fluid that is lost during the procedure.

Nucleus disassembly is broadly similar to techniques currently available, using either divide and conquer or phaco chop techniques, chopping being the favored method of most surgeons. Currently, the wound still needs to be enlarged to admit most types of implant, although some surgeons claim to be able to insert lenses through a 2.4-mm incision. Graham Barrett has recently described a technique called microcoaxial phaco, wherein a coaxial phaco probe is used that has just been reduced in size to 2.2 mm. He uses a modified sleeve and a standard microflow phaco needle, and can use an incision as small as 2 mm. This means that induced astigmatism is still negligible, but it does allow surgeons to carry on with techniques that are familiar to them, albeit with a smaller instrument.

Ultimately, when lenses are produced that will fold through a 1-mm incision, these techniques will become more important. Certainly, at present, microcoaxial phacoemulsification would seem to provide a similar advantage to the bimanual technique of microincision cataract surgery, while retaining the familiarity of standard phacoemulsification. Figure 9.17 shows microincision cataract surgery with the bimanual technique.

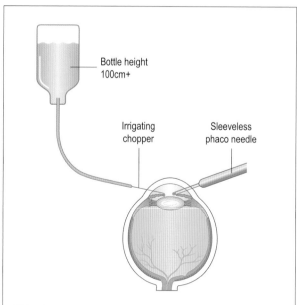

Bottle height
100cm+

Irrigating
chopper

Sleeveless
phaco needle

■ **FIGURE 9.17** Principles of microincision cataract surgery. Increased bottle height is required to maintain anterior chamber depth, due to leakage around the rigid irrigating chopper. The phaco probe is sleeveless because of technology that prevents heat buildup.

REFERENCES

1. Nagahara K. Phaco chop technique eliminates central sculpting and allows faster, safer phaco. Ocul Surg News 1993; October:12–13.
2. Koch PS. Stop chop phacoemulsification. J Cataract Refract Surg 1994; 20:566–570.
3. Dodick JM, Sperber LT, Lally JM, et al. Neodymium–YAG laser phacolysis of the human cataractous lens. Arch Ophthalmol 1993; 111(7):903–904.
4. Benjamin L. Laser phacoemulsification. Ophthalmol Pract 2001; 19(2):58–62.
5. Kanellopoulos AJ. Laser cataract surgery: a prospective clinical evaluation of 1,000 consecutive laser cataract procedures using the Dodick photolysis Nd-YAG system. Photolysis Investigative Group. Ophthalmology 2001; 108(4):649–654.

10

Irrigation–aspiration

The hard work is out of the way, and it is at this stage that complications such as vitreous loss often occur because of lack of concentration. This is an important part of the procedure and requires attention to detail, just as every other part of the operation. Two main methods of irrigation–aspiration are by using coaxial instruments or by separating the irrigation and aspiration, attached to separate instruments, the so-called bimanual technique.

COAXIAL IRRIGATION–ASPIRATION

A typical instrument is shown in Figure 10.1. Once nucleus removal has been completed, the irrigation and aspiration lines from the phaco machine are attached to the handpiece. The foot pedal now becomes a two-position instrument, with position 1 switching on the irrigation fluid and position 2 controlling the pump, in the case of a peristaltic machine in a linear fashion, and for a Venturi system, controlling the vacuum linearly. The instrument is introduced into the anterior chamber with the irrigation on, and the upward-facing port of the instrument is placed underneath the soft lens matter, which is itself underneath the anterior capsule. Position 2 of the foot pedal is applied, and the port on the instrument is blocked with soft lens matter, which causes a vacuum to rise. The soft lens matter can then be gently drawn into the middle of the anterior chamber, where increasing vacuum is applied to remove the soft lens matter. This process is repeated throughout 360°.

It can be difficult to get at the subincisional soft lens matter, especially if the capsulorrhexis is rather small, as the capsule inhibits access to the soft lens matter and has to be 'reached over'. This can be overcome by using a second tip on the irrigation–aspiration cannula, as shown in Figure 10.2. These aspiration tips vary in angle from 30 to 90° and make reaching subincisional cortical matter much easier. Some surgeons prefer to use a Simcoe cannula through a side port; this gives very good access to the subincisional cortex, but it is important only to enlarge the side port at the time of irrigation–aspiration, rather than at the

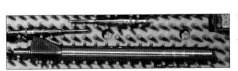

■ **FIGURE 10.1.** A typical irrigation–aspiration handpiece with two inter tips (interchangeable tips). These can be provided as one-piece instruments now.

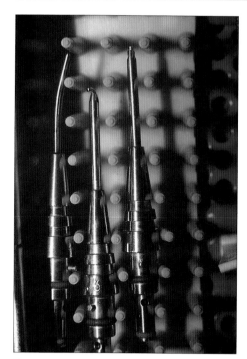

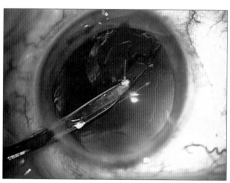

 FIGURE 10.3. The Simcoe cannula is gently curved and flattened in profile. The arrows show the outward flow of irrigation and the inward flow toward the aspiration port.

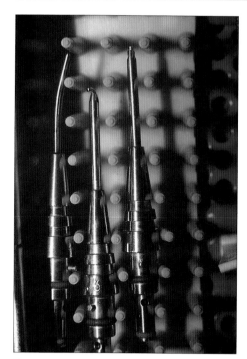 **FIGURE 10.2.** Three inter tips showing variable angle tips. The 90° tip shown in this picture is useful for reaching subincisional cortex.

beginning of the procedure, to accommodate the Simcoe, which is a large instrument. Otherwise, the anterior chamber will become unstable by losing a lot of fluid through this enlarged side port. Following complete removal of the soft lens matter, residual lens epithelial cells can be removed from the underside of the anterior capsule using the irrigation–aspiration tip. This can minimize the shrinkage of the capsulorrhexis opening.[1]

Simcoe cannula

This instrument was very popular in the days of extracapsular cataract surgery, and is still incredibly versatile in terms of giving access to the various areas under the capsulorrhexis, especially if used through an enlarged side port. Figure 10.3 shows the Simcoe cannula. Its gentle curve and flattened profile mean that it allows for a very stable anterior chamber, even when used for extracapsular surgery, and it is still favored by many surgeons. The side port needs to be considerably enlarged to admit this instrument into the eye, and enlargement of the side port must be made only at the time of irrigation–aspiration.

10.2

BIMANUAL IRRIGATION–ASPIRATION

Figure 10.4 shows a pair of bimanual irrigation–aspiration instruments, which come in different gauges and can be

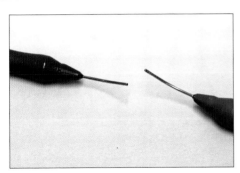

FIGURE 10.4. Bimanual disposable irrigation–aspiration instruments. They can be swapped between hands to achieve unparalleled access to cortex.

BOX 10.1 Removal of cortical soft lens matter

- Ensure deep chamber with continuous irrigation.
- Do not over-enlarge side ports.
- Keep aspiration port facing upward.

Subincisional cortex

- Do it first while bag open.
- Use angled aspiration tip (45°).
- Use two or more access sites.
- Separate irrigation–aspiration cannulae (bimanual).
- Engage SLM: allow vacuum to build up then pull centrally and aspirate in midchamber.

---

swapped between the right and left hands to give access to any part of the cortex. One of the instruments can be used through the main port, but this can lead to leakage of fluid around the instrument, therefore a separate side port is usually made. Box 10.1 shows a list of suggestions that can make removing the cortex safe and efficient.

REFERENCE

1. Hanson RJ, Rubinstein A, Sarangapani S, et al. Effect of lens epithelial cell aspiration on postoperative capsulorhexis contraction with the use of the Acnysot intraocular lens: randomized clinical trial. J Cataract Refract Surg 2006; 32:1621–1626.

11

Lens implantation and its history

HISTORICAL ASPECTS OF LENS IMPLANTATION

In November 1949, Harold Ridley at St Thomas's Hospital in London implanted the world's first intraocular lens. As with other great pioneering achievements, serendipity played a part in this fascinating story. Ridley noticed, as must a number of other people at the time, that when polymethyl-methacrylate (PMMA, perspex) was present as a foreign body in the human eye, it did not excite much of a reaction. His pioneering innovation was to make the link between this fact and the possibility of using perspex as an artificial lens following cataract surgery. The perspex in question had often come from the canopies of World War II fighter planes, which had shattered during battle and fragments of which had found their way into the eyes of pilots.

Ridley collaborated with Rayners in Hove, near Brighton on the south coast of England, in the design and manu-facture of the world's first implant, which was a biconvex disk of perspex. The original name for perspex was acrylic. In order for the implant to have a safe place to sit, Ridley utilized the extracapsular technique with a Graefe section, an anterior capsulectomy using a sharp cystotome and capsule forceps, before expressing the mature nucleus and washing out the anterior chamber. No gloves or micro-scopes were used, and Figure 11.1 shows stills from cine-matographic film taken of these first cases. High astigmatism and endothelial damage were not uncommon with this pro-cedure, but certainly some of the initial cases Ridley reported had initial good postoperative corrected visual acuity.

Unfortunately, a lack of knowledge (the function of the endothelium had not yet been described), the lack of micro-surgical tools and viscoelastics, and the lack of magnifica-tion that an operating microscope would have provided, as well as yet immature technique development (in the bag placement of the implant was virtually impossible to guarantee) all conspired against the development of lens implantation in the early days. Some of the early lenses were stored in centrimide, which actually absorbed into the PMMA substance and subsequently leaked into the fluid of the anterior chamber once implanted. This caused a uveitis, which was initially attributed to the lens material itself.

Having sustained a 20% failure rate for his initial im-plant surgery, Ridley abandoned the technique in 1964. The

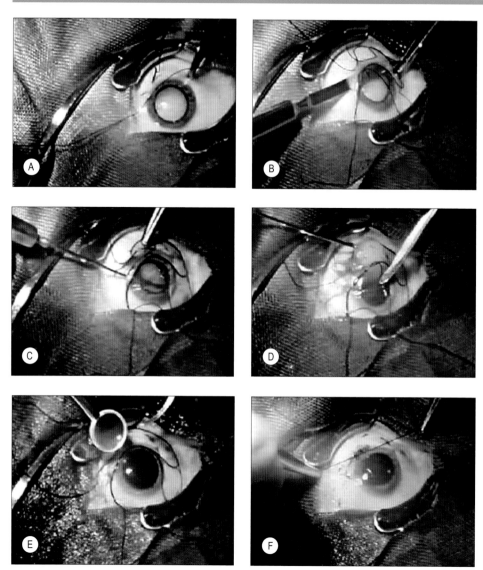

FIGURE 11.1 (**A**) A limbal silk suture being preplaced. (**B**) A Graefe knife being used ab interno to open the eye. A conjunctival flap is fashioned as the blade is drawn upward out of the eye. (**C**) A sharp cystotome is drawn across the anterior capsule to cut an opening in it. (**D**) Expression of the mature nucleus 'wheeled' out of the eye with a cystotome. (**E**) One of the world's first intraocular lens implants: a biconvex disk of polymethylmethacrylate. The lens had a groove around its edge to facilitate holding it during insertion. (**F**) The preplaced suture tied tightly across the wound.

main problem he was facing was finding a safe and secure way to place the implant without the attendant complications of dislocation, glaucoma, and others. Iris fixation was tried with a German design of lens, but this too failed to avoid the complications of corneal decompensation and bullous keratopathy. Further problems were described by Professor Barraque in Barcelona, who had to remove half of the 500 or so anterior chamber lenses he had implanted. The main issue was again that of bullous keratopathy. Peter Joyce in the UK persevered with nine different designs of anterior chamber lens over a period of 20 years or so, but some of the early models led to disastrous results.

Cornelius Binkhorst introduced the so-called iris clip lens in 1958, and although his initial design had four loops, two in front of the iris and two behind, he later abandoned the two anterior loops, finding that the implant was sufficiently stable with the optic in front of the iris and the two posterior haptics keeping it securely in place, as long as myotics were used to constrict the pupil.

Many designs of anterior chamber implant were tried, but because of deficiencies in manufacturing tolerances and quality control the vast majority were subsequently withdrawn. Tens of thousands of patients suffered adverse reactions to poorly designed and poor quality–controlled lenses during this period. In 1975, Sheerin designed J-shaped haptics on a PMMA optic, which became the forerunner of many extracapsular lenses designed to go in the capsular bag or the ciliary sulcus. Many modifications of this lens have been tried, but the most useful one was the forward angulation of the haptics introduced in 1980 by Richard Kratz.

The size of the optic became important with the increased usage of phacoemulsification small incision surgery, and initial experiments with hydrogel material were performed in 1976. Silicone was also tried, but so-called hydrophilic and hydrophobic acrylics (the original name for perspex was acrylic and the so-called modern acrylics are all modified molecules with different glass temperatures) have become increasingly popular.

Multifocal lenses have now also been introduced to combat the immediate presbyopia introduced by pseudophakia, and these are examined in more detail in Chapter 15 (*Lens exchange [including refractive lens exchange]*).

INTRAOCULAR LENS INSERTION

Intraocular lens insertion is what has made cataract surgery the success story it is today, by providing instant accurate visual rehabilitation. The operation provides patients with remarkable restoration of sight.

Although the optics of the human eye are complex, the history of implantation goes back to 1949, when, as described above, Harold Ridley started implanting lenses made of perspex. Subsequently, materials science has made it possible to use foldable implants through small incisions. The knowledge and application of aberrations relating to the eye is still a relatively young science. Significant perceived failure of the lens implantation operation can arise from an inappropriate or wrong-strength implant being used, and remains a significant source of patient and surgeon dissatisfaction.

The type of material from which the implant is made should be considered carefully. As yet, perspex is still the only substance with a very long track record (50 years). Pediatric implantation should therefore be carefully considered, as potentially these patients have several decades to live, and it is important to ensure that they have reliable, good-quality implants. Many hundreds of different lens styles and designs now exist, and careful assessment of a new implant is very important to ensure that it incorporates proven technology as well as tried and tested materials.

Posterior capsule opacification is a significant complication arising after cataract surgery in large numbers of patients, and puts them through an unnecessary, unpleasant episode of gradual visual loss again. Implants with a good track record of low posterior capsule opacification rates should therefore be sought.

Lens material and design seem to be important in preventing posterior capsule opacification, and it seems that hydrophobic acrylic as a material of choice, combined with a lens with a straight edge to the design, is best at preventing this. In the study by Auffarth et al., the European Posterior Capsular Opacification Study Group showed highly statistically significant differences between implant groups for the incidence of posterior capsular opacification and yttrium–aluminum–garnet (YAG) laser treatment.[1] Their mean delay for laser treatment from the date of cataract surgery was 2.48 years, ranging from 0 to 5.88 years, and the rates for YAG laser capsulotomy over the follow-up period were lowest in the hydrophobic acrylic group (7.1%), followed by silicone (16.2%), PMMA (19.3%), and hydrophilic acrylic (31.1%).

Other factors that need to be taken into account are, for example, the possible future use of silicone oil in the eye, which can emulsify the presence of a silicone lens and a posterior capsulotomy. A study by Abela-Formanek et al. showed the different biocompatibilities of lens materials to uveal and capsular tissue,[2] and these sorts of issue need to be carefully considered in patients with preexisting uveitis.

INSERTION TECHNIQUE

Wound enlargement

Most implants necessitate at least slight enlargement of the wound, and manufacturers make claims about the size of wound that their lenses will go through. A 3.5-mm wound is usually very stable, and a 4.5-mm wound is usually not. It is therefore very important to accurately enlarge the wound; this is best done by measuring the amount of enlargement. Most surgeons will enlarge the wound without measuring, and it is a useful exercise to ask several surgeons in a room to draw a line 3 mm long and then measure them accurately. In my experience, the resulting lines vary between 2 and 8 mm in size for inexperienced surgeons, and are more closely grouped for more experienced surgeons. It is therefore easy to over-enlarge the wound and make it unstable; therefore, by simply measuring the wound with a pair of calipers, this problem can be avoided. Once the type of implant has been decided, a set amount of enlargement can then be made each time the operation is performed. This should give repeatable and accurate wound enlargement.

Injectors

11.1

Figure 11.2A shows an injection cartridge and injector. Figure 11.2B and C shows the lens being folded into the cartridge, and the cartridge being placed into the injector before insertion into the eye. Injectors have the supposed advantage of the implant not touching the surface of the eye. However, the tip of the injector of course does touch the eye, but it is likely that the injector can be used via a smaller incision than with a folded implant. Most injectors have to be filled with viscoelastic in order to allow smooth passage of the lens through their lumen, and a variety of mechanisms exist to guide the implant down the lumen of the injector and into the eye in a controlled way. Figure 11.3 shows one such injector being used to deliver an implant into the anterior chamber under the protection of a viscoelastic. The lens is finally dialed into place with an instrument such as a Sinskey hook and positioned centrally in the capsular bag.

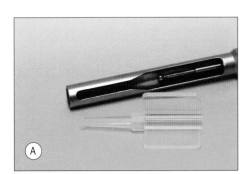

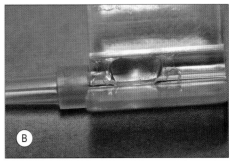

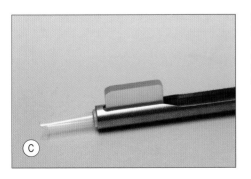

■ **FIGURE 11.2** (**A**) An injector and cartridge prior to loading the lens. (**B**) A plate haptic lens positioned in the cartridge before folding. (**C**) The cartridge is folded in half, positioned in the top of the injector, and inserted into the eye in the position shown, with bevel down.

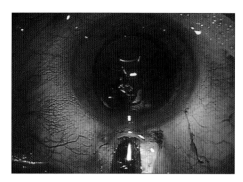

FIGURE 11.3 The injector in the eye with the lens beginning to unfold in the anterior chamber.

Folding forceps

Figure 11.4A shows a lens having been folded and placed into the lens forceps ready for delivery into the eye. Figure 11.4B and C shows insertion into the anterior chamber and the dialing in of the lens into position. The lens can be folded with the haptics either longitudinally or horizontally (Fig. 11.4D). The advantage of longitudinal folding is that the leading haptic can be inserted straight into the capsular bag and the trailing haptic dialed in subsequently. The stated advantage of folding the lens horizontally is that both legs can be placed into the central anterior chamber; as the lens unfolds, both legs unfold automatically into the capsular bag, under the anterior capsular edges. It is slightly more difficult to insert a lens folded horizontally, and care must be taken with lens materials that unfold rapidly, as the haptics can cause damage to the capsule if both spring apart forcibly once inside the eye. A number of lenses are manufactured with the haptics anteriorly vaulted; if this is the case, the lens should be injected such that it is able to be dialed clockwise, without the open end of the haptic coming into contact with the capsular bag. If this is not apparent, then the lens has been put in upside down and should be carefully manipulated into the right position. Figure 11.5A and B shows the correct and incorrect orientation of the lenses with respect to dialing.

Viscoelastic should be removed from the anterior chamber, and especially from behind the lens, as the effectivity of the implant can be changed by excess viscoelastic pushing it forward.

11.2
11.3

NON-FOLDING IMPLANTS

Figure 11.6 shows a solid PMMA lens being inserted into an eye having had an extracapsular cataract extraction. This is done using a McPherson's forceps, guiding the leading haptic into the capsular bag, and subsequently either dialing the lens into position or using a pair of forceps to guide the trailing haptic into the upper part of the capsular bag. It is

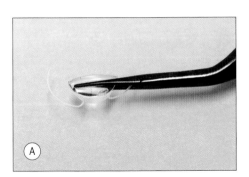
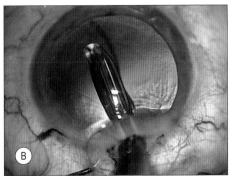
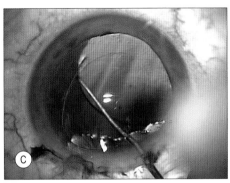
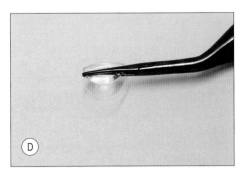

■ **FIGURE 11.4** (**A**) The traditional longitudinal method of folding an implant in forceps ready for delivery into the eye. The leading haptic can be placed straight into the capsular bag. (**B**) The lens during insertion, with the leading haptic in the bag. (**C**) The lens is dialed into position, ensuring that the trailing haptic is placed below the capsulorrhexis margin and into the capsular bag. (**D**) An alternative way of folding an implant, so that both haptics unfold into the bag at once. Folded this way, lenses can be slightly more difficult to insert, as they are more bulky and may need a slightly larger incision. There is also the risk with silicone lenses, which unfold rapidly, of capsular damage if controlled holding is not obtained.

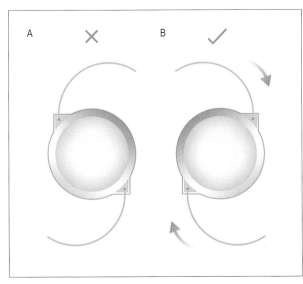

■ **FIGURE 11.5** Lenses are usually constructed so that the lens can be dialed clockwise once it is in the capsular bag, without the open ends of the haptics impinging on the capsule. If the lens is sitting as shown in (**A**), dialing it clockwise will snag the capsular bag and usually implies that the lens has been put in upside down. (**B**) Correct orientation, with the ability to dial clockwise.

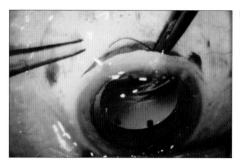

FIGURE 11.6 An intraocular lens being placed into the capsular bag through an extracapsular incision. Copious amounts of viscoelastic must be used to prevent endothelial damage.

important to use copious amounts of viscoelastic to ensure endothelial protection, as contact between the implant and the endothelium results in a huge loss of the endothelial cell population.

ANTERIOR CHAMBER IMPLANT

11.4

This is inserted using a McPherson's forceps, and it may be guided into the anterior chamber over a Sheets glide.[3] This is a sterile piece of plastic that is inserted through the cataract wound and in front of the iris, and guides the implant into position in the anterior chamber. The leading haptic can be placed relatively easily in the drainage angle opposite the wound, and the trailing haptic can be either pushed into position, using a Y-shaped pusher, or indeed pulled into position via the side port, using a dialing hook. It should then be manipulated so that the feet sit in the drainage angle and do not push peripheral iris into the angle. A sign that this has happened is a peaked pupil in the direction of the offending haptics. Gentle manipulations can lift the haptics off the iris and into the angle. In a patient with known glaucoma, or who is at risk of developing glaucoma, it is sensible to use a non–angle-supported lens.

IRIS-SUPPORTED LENS

The Artisan (Ophtec) is supported by enclavating or trapping some iris stromal tissue in a clawlike opening in the haptics of the lens. The lens has been designed for phakic use to correct myopia, but it is also a useful lens to use in aphakic eyes, although a little tricky to insert. Figure 11.7 shows an Artisan lens in place, and demonstrates the slight oblong peaking of the pupil that occurs due to the enclavation of the iris into the lens haptics. The figure shows a lens in position having been enclavated on to the iris stroma.

SUTURED POSTERIOR CHAMBER IMPLANTS

These implants are usually not folding and have an eyelet in each haptic, through which a suture can be passed. The needle on the sutures is then fed through the pupil and out

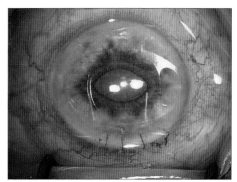

■ **FIGURE 11.7** An Artisan lens in place. The haptics of the lens have a split in them, and the iris is enclavated or trapped in between the claws of the lens. The pupil has been stretched slightly sideways by this technique. It is a good lens to use in patients with glaucoma, as it does not interfere with the drainage angle.

through the sclera around 3.5 mm from the limbus. The sutures hold the implant in place against the pars planar and require no capsular support. By using appropriate knots, ordinary folding implants can be used in this fashion, as long as the prolene sutures are secured well on to the haptics. There are, as yet, little data on the biocompatibility of such lenses used in this fashion.

IRIS-SUTURED IMPLANTS

A beautiful description of the iris-sutured implant is given in Bruce Noble's book.[4] The advantages of this technique are that the passage of a needle through the pars planar is avoided, and it can be combined with iris reconstruction, if required at the time.

MULTIFOCAL IMPLANTS

The optics of these lenses are described in more detail in a later chapter, but from the point of view of insertion into the eye they all demand very careful centration and as little tilt as possible to work effectively. Careful attention must be paid to the position site and size of the capsulorrhexis opening to allow full access of the optical zone of these implants so that they can be effective in providing multifocal vision. Clearly, a decentered lens with an eccentric capsulorrhexis, which is too small and then shrinks further, will have a deleterious effect on the multifocality of the implant. Similarly, careful consideration must be given to the wound construction in these patients, as leaving the corneal surface as spherical as possible is very important for these lenses to be effective. Careful astigmatically neutral surgery must be planned when these lenses are used. In terms of their folding and insertion into the eye, they are no different to other styles of foldable implant; some may be inserted with forceps and some through an injector system. Lens material and design are also important in terms of preventing posterior capsular opacification with these implants, as this will also markedly reduce their effectiveness.

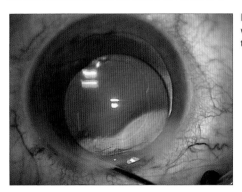

■ FIGURE 11.8 Stromal hydration ensures a secure wound as the patient is transferred from the operating table.

WOUND HYDRATION

If the wound has been carefully constructed and contains at least one step and two planes, then it should be self-sealing. A number of surgeons will hydrate the wound postoperatively to ensure that the wound is stable as the patient is moved from the operating table or chair back to the recovery area. Stromal hydration is accomplished by injecting balanced salt solution, via a 27-gauge cannula, into the stroma at the edge of the wound, as shown in Figure 11.8. Quite often, the edges of the wound are slightly unstable, as the wound has been enlarged to admit the implant, and the enlargement may not have been in the same orientation as the original valvelike wound. If there is any uncertainty as to the stability of the wound, it should be closed with a suture. A variety of these exist, but the so-called infinity suture is a very useful one to use.

SUBCONJUNCTIVAL INJECTION

An antibiotic and steroid combination is used in the subconjunctival space. The patient should be warned that this can be uncomfortable due to distension of the tissues. The eye is padded and covered with a shield, and the patient can be transferred to the recovery area.

REFERENCES

1. Auffarth GU, Brezin A, Caporossi A, et al. for the European PCO study group. Comparison of ND:YAG capsulotomy rates following phacoemulsification with implantation of PMMA, silicone or acrylic intraocular lenses in four European countries. Ophthalmic Epidemiol 2004; 11(4):319–329.
2. Abela-Formanek C, Amon M, Schauersberger J, et al. Results of hydrophilic acrylic, hydrophobic acrylic and silicone intraocular lenses in uveitic eyes with cataract: comparison to a control group. J Cataract Refract Surg 2002; 28(7):1141–1152.
3. Simcoe CW. Versatilitiy of the Sheets lens glide. J Am Intraocul Implant Soc 1983; 9(3):326.
4. Noble BA, Simmonds IG, Chang BYP. Anterior segment repair reconstruction techniques and medicolegal issues. London: Butterworth Heinemann; 2001.

12 Postoperative care

The end of the phacoemulsification or cataract procedure is the beginning of an important period of time for the patient. The eye is often padded and protected with a plastic shield immediately after the operation, for at least a few hours. In patients in whom the only good eye has been operated on, then it is reasonable to place a clear shield only over the eye, so that they have a degree of vision while recovering from the surgery.

After transfer back to the recovery area, the patient should be given clear instructions as to how to look after the eye postoperatively and what to expect in terms of vision, comfort, and visual rehabilitation. Clear instructions about the use of topical drops should also be given, and it is usual to use an antibiotic and steroid, either separately or in combination, four times a day for a minimum of 2 weeks. The preoperative assessment should have disclosed any difficulties that patients might have with instilling their own drops, but this should certainly be checked at the point before discharge.

USE OF NON-STEROIDAL ANTIINFLAMMATORIES

A systematic review by Sivaprasad et al. showed a positive effect of 0.5% ketorolac tromethamine ophthalmic solution on chronic cystoid macular oedema.[1] However, this study found that there was not enough evidence to show the effectiveness of non-steroidal antiinflammatory drugs (NSAIDs) in acute cystoid macular oedema prevention following cataract surgery. Three trials looking at the effect of NSAIDs on acute cystoid macular oedema were too heterogeneous to allow a metaanalysis, and therefore it is possible that there is a positive effect; certainly, if the patient has suffered cystoid macular oedema in one eye postoperatively, it is probably worth using steroids and NSAIDs postoperatively to try to prevent it occurring in the second eye.

INSTRUCTIONS

Written instructions are useful, as patients often do not remember the detail of what they are told at the time of surgery or shortly thereafter. These instructions should contain information about what to do and who to contact if the patient feels that things are not progressing satisfactorily, or if there are any sudden changes in symptomatology. Pain, increasing redness, and decreasing vision are the three cardinal symptoms that must be reported immediately, and the clinic or ward staff must be properly educated as to how to respond to a patient inquiring about such symptoms. The facility to review a patient with these symptoms immediately must be available. If it is not the surgeon who is contacted directly, then persons taking the phone call must have a degree of experience that allows them to make a judgment about whether the patient needs seeing immediately or can wait for a more routine appointment.

FURTHER ASSESSMENT

Assessment at 2 weeks postoperatively is useful, as, if the eye is quiet and comfortable at that stage, topical drops can be tapered fairly rapidly. However, if there are continuing signs of anterior segment inflammation, they may be continued at the full dose for a longer period. Refraction for glasses can be carried out at around 1 month, when the corneal wound will be stable, assuming that it has not been made larger than around 3.5 mm. If a stitch is in place, this should be removed before refraction is undertaken. A decision about cataract surgery in the second eye, if it has not been done, can be taken at this stage, and indeed may need to be contemplated fairly soon after the first eye if anisometropia exists. In the case of high myopes, it is sensible to book two dates fairly close together for the two operations, so that this period of inconvenience between the two eyes being done is minimized.

AUDIT AND OUTCOMES

Audit and outcomes are essential to ensure maintenance of standards of surgery, but also to ensure that measurements such as biometry are accurate, and that planned outcomes are achieved. Individualization of A constants for implants is possible, with a retrospective analysis of 50–100 implants by the same surgeon, and this should be undertaken to ensure that any particular surgical foibles are taken into account and corrected for. A number of outcome measures can be audited; these can guide issues such as continuing medical education, targeted retraining, or changes in technique, depending on their outcomes.

NATIONAL CATARACT AUDITS

In the UK, a national cataract data-set is being set up, which will allow comparisons between units across the country to be made. The data are anonymized and are returned centrally and analyzed. The outcome data are then returned to each individual unit, showing where they come on a national scale, and again can be informative about any particular aspect of the service that needs addressing.

Existing systems, such as the Swedish national database,[2] are very useful and allow units to monitor their outcomes with respect to nationally derived standards. The data can be made available down to the level of an individual surgeon. Again, because the data are anonymized, this allows surgeons to assess their outcomes against known standards. This can inform continued medical education or targeted training, if necessary.

PATIENT-BASED OUTCOMES

In our unit, we have developed and used a validated model for assessing visual outcomes after cataract surgery.[3] Such models are useful for assessing the impact of the service delivered to the local population.

REFERENCES

1. Sivaprasad S, Bunce C, Wormold R. Non-steroidal anti-inflammatory agents for cystoid macular oedema following cataract surgery: a systemic review. Br J Ophthalmol 2005; 89(11):1420–1422.
2. Lundstrom M, Stenevi U, Thorburn W. The Swedish National Cataract Register: a 9-year review. Acta Ophthalmol Scand 2002; 80:248–257.
3. Lawrence DJ, Brogan C, Benjamin L, et al. Measuring the effectiveness of cataract surgery: the reliability and validity of a visual function outcomes instrument. Br J Ophthalmol 1999; 83:66–70.

13

Adjuncts for and management of complex cases

SMALL PUPIL

There are a number of strategies for dealing with small pupils. These include iris hooks, pupil stretching, the Perfect Pupil device, and high molecular weight viscoelastics. Each has its advantages and disadvantages, which will be discussed.

High molecular weight viscoelastic

Healon 5 (AMO) has a molecular weight of 5 million Daltons and is a so-called viscoadaptive viscoelastic (see Ch. 6). It is very useful for moving tissues, and will maintain a deep anterior chamber as well as encourage and cause pupil mydriasis when injected into the anterior chamber. Sometimes, the pupil can be expanded from 2 or 3 mm up to 4 or 5 mm, which is an adequate size for safe phacoemulsification. Healon GV (greater viscosity) (AMO) can also be used but has a lower molecular weight (4 million Daltons) and is less effective at tissue separation.

Iris hooks

These come in sets of either four or five and consist of a polypropylene hook with a rubber or plastic stop, which can be used to retract and hold the iris or capsule (Fig. 13.1). They are inserted through a paracentesis, which is made in a relatively flat plane at the limbus. If these wounds are made too steeply, then the hook has the effect of tenting the

13.1

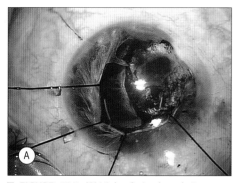
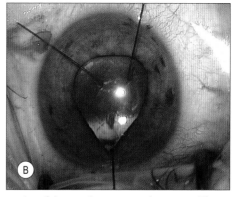

■ **FIGURE 13.1 (A)** Iris hooks in place during a reconstruction of the anterior segment after trauma. The hooks have a stop, which is slid down the length of the hooks to keep them in place. **(B)** Iris hooks used to open the pupil but also to stabilize the capsular bag during phacoemulsification in a subluxed lens.

iris upward toward the cornea (Fig. 13.2). Four hooks are usually inserted and give a square pupil, but of an adequate size that a 4- to 5-mm capsulorrhexis can be constructed within the confines of the enlarged pupil. The hooks are also useful for stabilizing the capsular bag once the rhexis has been fashioned, and it is possible to use eight hooks, four for the iris and four for the capsular bag, to keep things stable while the operation continues. Where there is capsular instability, and this is necessary, a slow-flow set of phaco parameters are used. This means a low bottle height, slow aspiration rate, and low vacuum, with low phaco power and gentle manipulations of the nucleus. The hooks are removed at the end of the procedure by sliding the locking collar toward the free end of the hook, and gently pushing the hook centrally into the anterior chamber before depressing the free end to lift the hook clear of the iris, at which point it can be pulled out of the eye. If it is simply pulled straight out from its position over the iris edge, then it is not unusual to get pigment pulled out with it, which gets trapped in the paracentesis. Figure 13.3 shows hook removal.

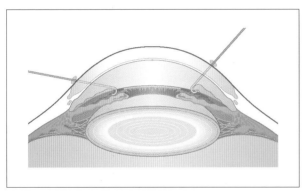

■ **FIGURE 13.2** Tenting up of the iris if the hook is positioned too steeply through the cornea.

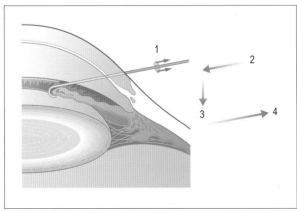

■ **FIGURE 13.3** Removal is carried out by first sliding the locking collar up the shaft of the hook (1). A pair of non-toothed forceps is then used to hold the protruding tip of the hook and push it inward (2) and downward (3), which lifts the hook into the anterior chamber and then outward (4). This removes the hook from the anterior chamber atraumatically.

Pupil stretching

Various instruments have been devised to stretch the pupil in two directions, vertically and horizontally, to tear the pupil sphincter and allow a mid-dilated pupil. This technique can work well but is quite traumatic for the iris and does involve partial rupture at least of the pupil sphincter. Figure 13.4 shows pupil stretching being performed. Although it is relatively quick and straightforward, it probably causes more breakdown of the blood–aqueous barrier than iris hooks do. A paracentesis is made at 3 and 9 o'clock, and the instruments inserted opposite one another cause a horizontal stretch. Then a pushing instrument is inserted through the phaco wound, and a pulling instrument inserted similarly through the phaco wound, to cause the vertical stretch. Care must be taken not to damage the corneal endothelium peripherally in the extremes of the manipulation of the iris.

Other devices

The Perfect Pupil (Becton Dickinson Ophthalmic Surgical, Waltham, Massachusetts) is a polymethylmethacrylate device inserted through the phaco wound and positioned within the pupil margin (Fig. 13.5). It dilates the pupil up to a preset size and allows a reasonable size capsulorrhexis within its borders. Pupil expansion up to approximately 8 mm can be obtained, and it is removed after surgery.[1] Significant

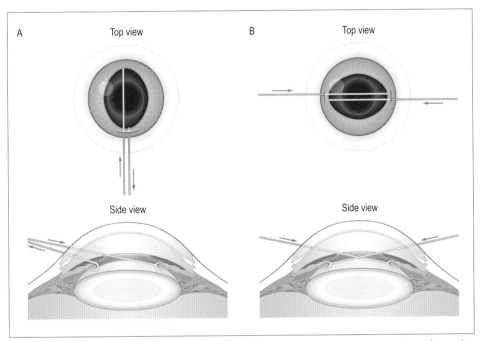

■ **FIGURE 13.4** A method for stretching the iris with two instruments. (**A**) One instrument is used to push and one to pull the iris. (**B**) Both instruments are placed via paracentesis at 3 and 9 o'clock, and both instruments push the iris.

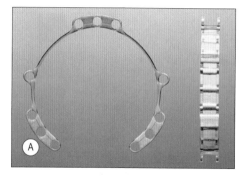

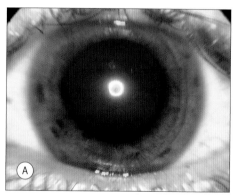

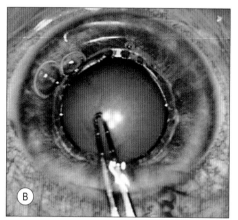

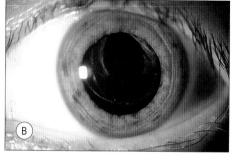

■ **FIGURE 13.5 (A)** The Perfect Pupil device inserted through a phaco wound and positioned within the pupillary margin helps to maintain it at a fixed diameter. **(B)** The device inside the eye during a capsulorrhexis.

■ **FIGURE 13.6 (A)** A dislocated crystalline lens. This lens is dislocated upward, as would be seen typically in Marfan syndrome. **(B)** The same lens postoperatively, with a capsular tension ring in the periphery of the bag, helping to centralize the bag to a degree. This capsular bag–lens complex needed a maneuver later to centralize it further, using a suture over the lens haptic through the edge of the capsular bag and out through the sclera.

traction on the iris root can be caused if the pupil device is inserted incorrectly, and care must be taken during removal not to damage the endothelium around the phaco wound.

Zonular support

Capsular tension rings are incredibly useful for supporting areas of lax zonular support. Figure 13.6 shows such a case pre- and postoperatively. The tension rings can be introduced after the capsulorrhexis is performed, into the peripheral cortical subcapsular region, but this produces significantly more stress on the zonules during surgery. It is easier to remove the cataract, if there is enough zonular support, and after irrigation–aspiration insert the capsular tension ring to centrate the capsular bag and support the weak quadrant. Modified rings, such as those designed by Cionni in Cincinnati,[2] can be used when there is significantly more than 180° of zonular weakness, for example in

Marfan syndrome. These rings have an eyelet through which a suture can be passed to centrate the tension ring–capsular bag complex after the insertion of the tensioning device. Insertion of a normal tension ring can be performed manually with two pairs of forceps, or via an injector, but should be commenced in such a way that further stress is not placed on the area of weak zonules. The tension rings are left in place after the surgery permanently. If the rings are inserted before the cataract is removed, then getting the cortical soft lens matter out can be more tricky. Instead of pulling the soft lens matter centrally into the safe zone of the anterior chamber, the lens matter is rather moved circumferentially around the ring until it is loose enough to be aspirated. Again, care must be taken not to stress the weakened area of zonule deficiency. The rings can be injected or fed into the capsular bag using non-toothed forceps. They remain in the eye permanently.

PSEUDOEXFOLIATION

Pseudoexfoliation may present no problems at all. However, unless the crystalline lens is frankly loose, anticipating trouble in each case is a good way to prevent problems. Capsulorrhexis will give a good indication as to the stability of the capsular bag–zonule complex. If excess movement of the complex is observed during the capsulorrhexis, very careful hydrodissection should be carried out. Viscoexpression using a U-shaped cannula is a useful maneuver to gently elevate the nucleus out of the bag with minimal zonular stress. 'Slow motion' phaco is a good method to adopt; essentially, this involves lowering the bottle height, slowing the aspiration rate, reducing the phaco power, and making small slow movements in the eye with all instruments. Any forward displacement of the bag–zonule complex during phacoemulsification should alert the surgeon to make slower, shallower movements with the probe. As longer episodes of phacoemulsification may be required to remove the lens because slow shallow movements are being made, careful attention to irrigation must be given to ensure that wound burns are avoided. If zonular dehiscence is noticed, the use of a capsule tension ring should be considered.

The use of the soft shell technique using a cohesive and dispersive viscoelastic should be considered, as the phacoemulsification may take longer than usual and endothelial protection is important. As these eyes are prone to develop glaucoma, avoidance of a postoperative pressure spike is important. Preservative-free antihypertensive agents can be administered topically at the end of the procedure or acetazolamide given orally for one or two nights after the operation.

If coexistent glaucoma is present, consideration may be given to a combined phaco–trabeculectomy procedure.

FUCH'S ENDOTHELIAL DYSTROPHY

The approach for these patients depends on the functional reserve of the endothelium. Normal corneal clarity can usually be maintained with cell counts above $1000/mm^2$. If diurnal variation in vision has been described, with blurring in the mornings and improved acuity as the day progresses, then the cell count is often below this level and can be expected to decompensate after any intraocular procedure, which threatens further endothelial cell loss. In these cases, combined penetrating keratoplasty and cataract extraction (usually by the extracapsular method once the eye is open) are recommended. If endothelial function is adequate, it is worthwhile attempting phacoemulsification. Assessment of endothelial function should include measurement of corneal thickness (pachymetry) in the morning. Measurements outside the expected normal range should be regarded as suspicious for decreased endothelial reserve. A figure of more than 0.6 mm should be regarded as indicating a functionally compromised corneal endothelium (assuming the cornea to have been normal thickness to begin with).

Alterations to technique for a case in which there is limited endothelial reserve include the following.

- Scleral tunnel wound to limit endothelial cell loss.
- Soft shell technique with viscoelastic to protect endothelium during phacoemulsification.
- Slow-motion phaco with reduced fluid flow and lower phaco power.
- Chop technique for more rapid nuclear disassembly.
- Phaco-assisted aspiration to remove as much nucleus as possible.
- Use of warm irrigation fluid.
- Avoidance of intracameral agents as far as possible.
- Avoidance of postoperative pressure spike.

Although there is evidence that carrying out a penetrating keratoplasty first, allowing the donor cornea time to stabilize optically, and then carrying out cataract surgery gives more predictable results, there are sustainable arguments for triple procedures (penetrating keratoplasty with extracapsular cataract extraction and intraocular lens insertion) to be carried out too.[3,4]

TRAUMATIC CATARACT

The timing of cataract removal after trauma can be difficult. It is often counterproductive to remove the lens at the time of a primary repair, for several reasons. First, working on a soft eye with an unstable anterior and/or posterior segment that may be bleeding from the iris or choroid is especially difficult. Second, traumatic cataract can be surprisingly compatible with reasonable vision once the eye settles after trauma repair. Finally, visualization of all the necessary structures may be impossible. Having said that, if a lens is completely disrupted and lens proteins are 'fluffing up' (hydrating) in the anterior chamber, a lens aspiration can sometimes be safely performed if the eye is closed and stable.

Trauma surgery necessitates preparation, planning, and an ability to think on one's feet and change a surgical plan, perhaps several times during a procedure, depending on the findings made intraoperatively.

Clearly, thorough preoperative evaluation must be undertaken following primary repair of the globe, and investigations such as B-scan ultrasound, computed tomography or magnetic resonance imaging, and others can help to acquire a full clinical picture.

The timing of reconstructive surgery may be influenced by many factors, such as the patient's age (early intervention in children to prevent amblyopia), the state of health of the patient (multiple injuries may preclude ideal timing), and associated eye injuries (repair of a retinal detachment may require early removal of a cataract).

Factors affecting surgery

These are as follows.

- The view of the anterior chamber may be partly obscured by sutured corneal wounds.
- There may be vitreous in the anterior chamber at the start of surgery.
- Iris tissue may be missing or trapped in the corneal wound.
- The anterior capsule may have been breached.
- There may be abnormal adhesions between tissue planes.

These and many other factors make the surgery unpredictable, technically demanding, and time-consuming. These cases should never be 'fitted in' but must be allocated sufficient time and facilities for safe surgery to be performed.

Copious use of viscoelastics is recommended throughout the procedure; this allows the delicate separation of tissues, hemostasis, maintenance of surgical space and planes, and endothelial protection. High molecular weight viscoelastics are very useful in cases with bulging anterior chambers.

When suturing corneal wounds, it is useful to gain primary closure with the use of slipknots and subsequently replace them with square (reef) knots at known tension. Practice knot tying in the skills laboratory is universally taught in the UK, as it has become less commonly observed since the virtual abandonment of extracapsular surgery through a large wound.

Figure 13.7 shows various steps in the primary repair and subsequent cataract surgery carried out on the eye of a 6-year-old boy who was hit in the eye by a stick while playing sword fighting with a friend in his garden. The initial repair was undertaken in the evening as the child was inconsolable. No preoperative x-rays or scans could

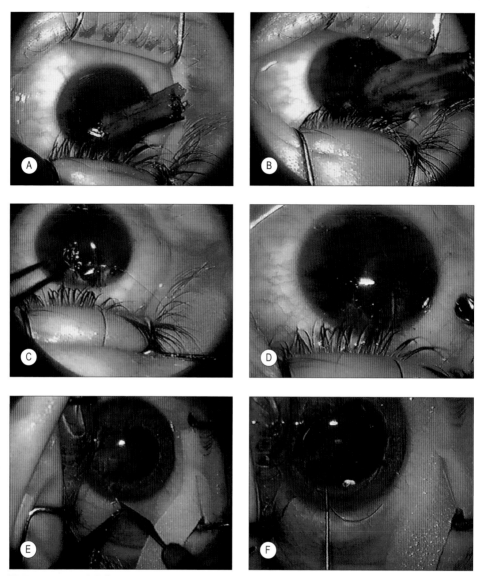

■ **FIGURE 13.7** (**A**) The original injury, showing entry of the wooden stick via the peripheral cornea. (**B**) The stick being gently withdrawn after copious lubrication with viscoelastic. Slightly enlarging the entry wound with a sharp blade can facilitate removal of rough-edged objects. The stick was sent for microbiology, as unusual organisms may be inoculated into the eye at the time of injury. (**C**) Primary wound closure with 10/0 nylon. (**D**) The wound at the end of primary closure, showing an almost total hyphema. (**E**) The start of cataract removal some weeks later via a temporal wound. Some iris tissue is missing superiorly. (**F**) Lens implantation against the posterior capsule was possible as, remarkably, it was mainly intact. Biometry of the fellow eye was undertaken as a check against the k readings of the warped, injured cornea and difficult technical measurement of axial length.

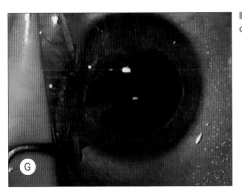

■ **FIGURE 13.7** (**G**) The eye at the end of the cataract removal.

be carried out, and the stick was carefully removed under general anesthesia. The corneal wound was sutured with 10/0 nylon. No anterior chamber details could be seen as it was full of blood, and the amount of lens involvement could not be ascertained.

Over the next few days as the eye settled, ultrasound provided evidence of a flat retina and an otherwise intact globe.

In view of the boy's age, cataract surgery was carried out relatively early. The lens had completely opacified within 24 h of the injury.

No capsular dye was available at the time, although nowadays it would be very useful to delineate the remaining capsule, which was remarkably intact. The surgery was relatively uneventful, and a posterior chamber lens was positioned within the capsular bag. Some iris sphincter damage was evident at the 12 o'clock position.

Subsequently, the patient underwent an yttrium–aluminum–garnet laser capsulotomy and today achieves 20/30 (6/9) visual acuity with the aid of a contact lens. If his surgery was being carried out today, consideration would be given to the use of a multifocal, aspheric intraocular lens implant to maximize his binocular capability for near and distance.

Summary

Trauma surgery and the management of traumatic cataract are time-consuming and highly variable. A complete range of surgical tools and a flexible approach need to be maintained.

POSTREFRACTIVE SURGERY INTRAOCULAR LENS CALCULATIONS

As the degree of flattening of the corneal surface is altered by laser refractive surgery, the standard keratometry readings cannot be used in biometry for cataract surgery. If they are used, a large hypermetropic error will ensue. There is no absolutely failsafe way of overcoming this, but two methods may be used that will give reasonable approximations. The first method is the contact lens method. This is the less accurate one. It is performed by refracting the patient with and without a plano-powered contact lens of known back surface power. The corrected keratometry value is obtained by the following formula:

contact lens (back surface power) + refraction (over contact lens) – refraction (without contact lens).

The refraction is then corrected for back vertex distance.

The second and more accurate method is the prior data method, which requires:

- the prerefractive surgery refraction and keratometry, and
- the postrefractive surgery refraction once the result has stabilized.

An example using this method follows.

Pre–photorefractive keratectomy (PRK) refraction
$$= -6.00 \text{ D}$$
Pre-PRK keratometry = 45 + 47 D (mean = 46 D)
Post-PRK refraction = −1.00 D
Change in refraction = −5.00 D
Mean k reading to use in intraocular lens calculation
$$= 46 - 5 = 40 \text{ D}.$$

Whichever method is used, the patient should be counseled that the result is an approximation and that future adjustment may be necessary.

INTRAOPERATIVE FLOPPY IRIS SYNDROME (IFIS)

This syndrome is brought about by patients taking tamsulosin, an α_{1A}-adrenoreceptor blocker, and other such drugs. During the course of phaco surgery, the iris diaphragm is floppy and has a tendency to billow out of the phaco wound and/or side ports. The iris sphincter tends to constrict during surgery.

To counteract this problem, advice about stopping the drug 2 weeks before surgery may be given, but this course of action may not be effective in all patients. The use of high molecular weight viscoelastics can help, but of most use seems to be the intracameral injection of dilute, preservative-free phenylephrine. This helps to keep the pupil dilated and seems to splint the iris during surgery. A low-flow infusion of fluid is also helpful. The phenylephrine can be made up by using 0.1 mL of preservative-free 2.5% phenylephrine and diluting this to 1 mL with balanced salt solution. Also useful is the placement of iris hooks to stabilize the iris if IFIS is encountered.

Other agents have been reported to be associated with intraoperative floppy iris syndrome, and animal studies have shown that several α_1-adrenoceptor antagonists affect normal iris dilatation tone. These include alfuzosin, doxazosin, naftopidil, prazosin, tamsulosin, and terazosin. This may indicate a class effect for this group of medicines.[5]

REFERENCES

1. Kershner RM. Management of the small pupil for clear corneal cataract surgery. J Cataract Refract Surg 2002; 28(10):1826–1831.
2. Cionni RJ, et al. Modified capsular tension ring for patients with congenital loss of zonular support. J Cataract Refract Surg 2003; 29(9):1668–1673.
3. Davis EA, Stark WJ. The triple procedure—is it the best approach for the patient? The triple procedure may be superior to sequen-tial surgery. Arch Ophthalmol 2000; 118(3):414–415.
4. Hamill MB. Sequential surgery may be the best approach for the patient. Arch Ophthalmol 2000; 118:415–417.
5. Michel MC, Okutsu H, Noguchi Y, et al. In vivo studies on the effects of α_1-adrenoceptor antagonists on pupil diameter and urethral tone in rabbits. Naunyn-Schmiedebergs Arch Pharmacol 2006; 372(5):346–353.

14

Management of complications

Complications will occur. It is hoped that as experience accrues, they occur less frequently and with fewer serious implications. The immediate management of complications may significantly alter the final outcome of a procedure and, because it is often the person who has caused the complication (the surgeon) who has to deal with it, it is most important that when a complication arises, the environment is conducive to continued, careful work, such that a good outcome is obtained. A supportive, efficient atmosphere should be maintained, and it does no harm, immediately after a complication (such as a vitreous loss), for the surgeon to sit back for a minute or so and review the surgical plan, and call for the relevant equipment in a calm and non-threatening voice, to re-establish the inner calm that is necessary for a successful surgery.

If a junior surgeon in training has caused a complication, then it is important that the trainer assesses the situation carefully. If the trainee still has reasonable confidence, the patient is comfortable and cooperative, and time allows, then complication management can be a very useful training exercise. Careful supervision is of course important, and it is equally important to use language in such a way that it does not frighten the patient or the trainee. For example, instead of saying 'No, don't do that', the phrase 'An alternative approach might be...' is more constructive and less threatening. There is no doubt that complications cause stress for all concerned, but careful management can produce good outcomes and good training.

At the point where further equipment is requested, it is very useful to have a member of the team holding the patient's hand and to distract the patient's attention from the proceedings by gently talking or chatting with her or him. Phrases from the hand-holder such as 'You are doing really well Mr(s) Smith; are you still reasonably comfortable on the operating table?' are useful distractions that can be used. It is also sometimes worthwhile for the surgeon to say to the patient something along the lines of 'We are going to be a few minutes more; are you still comfortable?' 'Would you like the music changed?' is another useful phrase.

Discussion of complications should take place relatively soon after the surgery, and an honest and straightforward account of what happened, what the implications are, and how future management will be handled should be given by the surgeon concerned. This approach will often be all that is required to reassure patients that their future care is in hand and allow them to ask any questions they might have.

PREOPERATIVE COMPLICATIONS
Local anesthesia
The main serious complication of sharp needle local anesthesia is perforation of the globe.[1] This can be avoided by asking the patient to look side to side once the needle is inserted, and if the globe is tethered at all then the needle should be withdrawn. Penetration of the globe is often accompanied by pain and resistance to injection, as the pressure in the globe rises. This also causes severe pain for the patient. If perforation is suspected, the needle should be gently withdrawn immediately, and the fundus inspected carefully with an indirect ophthalmoscope. Any sign of perforation should be treated by a vitreoretinal surgeon and may simply require cryotherapy to the perforation site, or more complicated measures if hemorrhage and/or detachment of the retina occur.

Peribulbar hemorrhage
Puncture of an orbital vessel is also often accompanied by pain, and gentle withdrawal of the syringe plunger should be carried out, before injection of local anesthetic is given, to ensure that the needle is not in the intraluminal compartment of a vessel. If a peribulbar hemorrhage occurs at the time of the local anesthetic administration, it is usual to abandon the procedure at that point, as increased bleeding can cause complications during surgery.

INTRAOPERATIVE COMPLICATIONS
Some of these are dealt with in their relevant chapters (e.g. capsule problems). The complications that will be discussed here are:
- the sudden hard eye,
- wound burn,
- dropped nucleus, and
- vitreous loss.

The sudden hard eye
There are two extraocular and three intraocular causes of a sudden hard eye perioperatively. A diagnostic cascade should be gone through if the eye suddenly becomes hard during the operation to determine a cause and thus an effective remedy (Fig. 14.1).

Extraocular causes
- Peribulbar hemorrhage can increase during the operation, and cause sudden pressure on the globe, which can make the eye feel very hard and shallow the anterior chamber. During this process, the iris usually prolapses from the wound, and the anterior chamber is completely

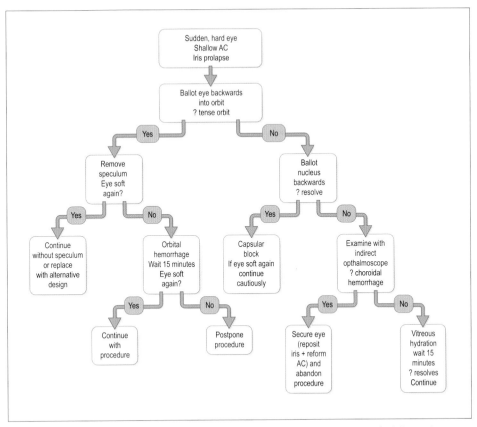

■ FIGURE 14.1 Algorithm for the management of a suddenly hard eye perioperatively. AC, anterior chamber.

lost. If an obvious orbital hemorrhage is visible, this makes a diagnosis, and it is worth tamponading the orbit temporarily to try to stop the bleeding, and subsequently to reform the anterior chamber, reposit the iris, and close the eye safely.

■ Pressure from the speculum. Sometimes the orbit is rather tight, and pressure from the lid speculum can raise the intraocular pressure, causing the same loss of anterior chamber and iris prolapse. Simply by manipulating the speculum, this factor can be reversed and pressure removed from the globe quickly.

Intraocular causes
■ Forcible injection of balanced salt solution (BSS) into the anterior chamber can cause a sudden movement of fluid through the zonules and into the anterior vitreous compartment, causing hydration of the vitreous and sudden hardening of the eye. This will usually sort itself out in 15 or 20 min, if left to its own devices, as the aqueous is reabsorbed and the situation resolves.

- Capsular block syndrome. This was referred to in Chapter 8 on hydrodissection, and occurs when a small capsulorrhexis is performed over a hard nucleus. Forcible injection of BSS into the capsular bag elevates the nucleus and causes it to block the capsulorrhexis, causing further distension posteriorly of the capsular bag. This can cause a sudden hardening of the eye and prolapse of the iris, with shallowing of the anterior chamber. By gently balloting the nucleus backward, this situation can often be reversed, but if it is not observed and continued injection of fluid occurs, then the posterior capsule can rupture, and pupil snap will be observed.
- Choroidal hemorrhage. With small-incision cataract surgery, expulsive hemorrhage is rare, but choroidal hemorrhage is probably more common than is expected. The eye becomes suddenly hard, the chamber is lost, and the iris prolapses. If all other causes have been excluded, it is worth looking into the eye with an indirect ophthalmoscope to see if a choroidal hemorrhage can be observed. If it can, the eye should not be further manipulated until the bleeding has tamponaded itself, and the eye should be left in this state for a few minutes. Following this, it is sometimes possible to reform the anterior chamber gently with viscoelastic, reposit the iris and, at that point, the situation should be left and the operation abandoned. Choroidal hemorrhages have been reported to occur in two phases, with the initial hardening of the eye, which then resolves, and a further more aggressive hemorrhage occurring after further manipulations of the globe have taken place. Sometimes the operation can be finished successfully, but it is probably safer to abandon the surgery and allow the eye to settle with topical antibiotic and steroid, and to reoperate after a few days. Figure 14.1 shows an algorithm for assessing a suddenly hard eye perioperatively, and this can be useful in diagnosing the cause before attempting to rectify it.

Wound burn

The main risk factors for a wound burn are a hard nucleus and a long corneal tunnel. Figure 14.2 shows the effect of a long corneal tunnel, with dimpling of the cornea, restriction of flow down the irrigating sleeve by compression in the tunnel, and angulation of the phaco probe on to the cataract and subsequent heat buildup. Ensuring a correct size and correct length tunnel can obviate this problem. A hard cataract can cause a problem, as when nuclear fragments occlude the tip of the phaco probe; if the needle is still vibrating in foot position 3, with the tip of the needle blocked, there is no significant flow of irrigating fluid to cool the needle. If this carries on for any length of time, the temperature of the needle and the wound can rise dramatically, causing tissue shrinkage and the wound to burn. The risk of this can be reduced by using modes such as

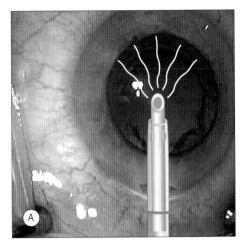 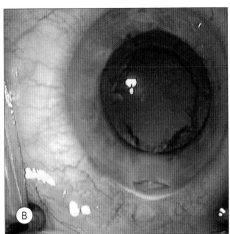

■ **FIGURE 14.2 (A)** Problems caused by a long corneal tunnel, with dimpling of the cornea due to angulation of the phaco probe, poor access to the superior part of the cataract, and poor irrigation due to pinching of the irrigation sleeve through the long tunnel and the angulation of the probe. **(B)** A wound burn due principally to the length of the corneal tunnel. Note how the anterior lip has shrunk away from the posterior lip.

pulsed or burst, which break up the phaco energy, but also by ensuring that nuclear fragments are as far as possible aspirated, and by using phacoemulsification only when absolutely necessary. This reduces the total energy in the eye and considerably reduces the risk of a wound burn.

If a wound burn does occur, the operation can continue as long as the cause of the burn is identified and dealt with. An infinity or cross-stitch can be used to close the burn wound, but it is important not to try to oppose the anterior and posterior lips of the wound in a vertical sense. The suture should be used just to close the wound in an antero-posterior direction, because if attempts are made to pull the shrunken anterior lip of the wound up to the posterior lip, significant astigmatism will be induced. Postoperatively, the burned cornea can sometimes recover remarkably well and heal with no significant problems, but if the burn is very significant, further measures, such as arcuate keratotomy, may be necessary to reduce the astigmatism induced by the surgery. Most phaco machines have a warning sound built in that indicates tip occlusion, and a new surgeon should be familiar with this sound. When it is heard, steps should be taken to reduce the occlusion to as short a time as possible, or limit the use of phaco power during the occlusion.

Dropped nucleus

It is important to have the discussion about management for a dropped nucleus with the vitreoretinal surgical collea-gues who would manage the case. If the surgeon concerned has vitreoretinal experience, then a primary retrieval of the dropped nucleus can be undertaken using a pars planar vitrectomy. Under no circumstances should attempts be made to elevate the nuclear fragment with the phaco probe. Indeed, as soon as any vitreous appears in the anterior chamber, the phaco probe needs to be carefully withdrawn, as it can induce very high vacuums and, by applying traction to the vitreous in this way, can cause a retinal detachment. Techniques have been described to elevate the fallen nucleus with the phaco probe, but only after a vitrectomy has been performed.

The reason for knowing the habits of the vitreoretinal surgeon are that there are two main methods of nucleus retrieval. The first involves a pars planar vitrectomy and the use of perfluorocarbon heavy liquid to elevate the nuclear fragment and retrieve it via the anterior segment, in which case an intraocular lens should not be implanted at the time of the primary procedure.[2] The second common way of removing the nuclear fragment is to carry out a pars planar vitrectomy and, using the fragmatome, emulsification of the nucleus can take place in the posterior segment. Again, perfluorocarbon may be used to float the nuclear fragment into mid vitreous cavity, or following as complete as possible vitrectomy, the fragmatome is introduced and vacuum used to elevate the fragments from the retina for them to be emulsified in the posterior segment. Either way, under these circumstances an implant can be used in a primary operation, as the fragments do not enter the anterior segment with this method. The timing of this surgery is important, and if there are significant nuclear fragments in the posterior segment, they should be removed within 5 days. By leaving them for longer periods of time, significant uveitis can occur, with consequent pressure problems and even retinal detachment.

The outcome of retrieval of nuclear fragments can be excellent, but the primary management is important in terms of ensuring that the anterior segment is dealt with adequately, by removal of vitreous and residual soft lens matter, paving the way for a reasonably quiet eye and a reasonable view for the vitreoretinal surgeon.

Vitreous loss

The incidence of vitreous loss during cataract surgery varies with experience and with the type of surgery. A number of the risk factors can be anticipated preoperatively, such as small pupils, subluxed lenses, the existence of pseudoexfoliation syndrome, previous blunt trauma, and uncooperative patients, and in some cases it is clearly iatrogenic. However, other factors, such as pre-existing unreported injuries or congenital zonular weakness, or anomalies, can also predispose to vitreous loss.

As this is the most common of the serious complications that occur intraoperatively, its management at the time of surgery is critical to the outcome of the particular case. Leaving vitreous in the anterior chamber and the wound can cause significant postoperative problems—from the more minor cosmetically peaked pupil to the more serious chronic cystoid macular edema and retinal detachment.

The principles of management of vitreous loss are to secure, as far as possible, the remaining nuclear and cortical fragments in the anterior segment, prevent further loss, and clear vitreous from the anterior segment and the front third of the vitreous cavity. It is imperative that if vitreous loss occurs during phacoemulsification, the phaco needle is stopped from vibrating immediately and the probe gently withdrawn from the eye, after ensuring that no vitreous has been aspirated into the needle lumen. The temptation to continue phacoing the vitreous must be avoided, as the phaco needle is very poor at cutting vitreous and simply acts as a large-bore aspirating needle applying high levels of traction to the vitreoretinal interface.

Having removed the phaco probe from the eye, an assessment of the situation takes place, and any obvious vitreous in the anterior segment can be removed with a vitreous cutter, usually set at the maximum cut rate. Some surgeons prefer to use a sleeved cutter with an integral coaxial infusion, and some prefer to separate the infusion from the cutter and use either an anterior chamber maintainer (Figure 14.3) or a separate infusion cannula admitted through the side port. The advantage of this is that the vitreous cutter is much finer without an irrigation sleeve, and will produce less edema of the phaco wound. A second paracentesis is sometimes made to admit the vitreous cutter, avoiding the self-sealing phaco wound altogether. Once any obvious vitreous has been removed from the anterior segment, any remaining nuclear or cortical fragments can be removed either with a vitreous cutter or with the phaco probe, as long as there is no sign of vitreous in the operating field. A recently described technique using triamcinolone in the anterior segment is excellent at identifying vitreous in the anterior chamber.[3] Figure 14.4 shows triamcinolone

14.1

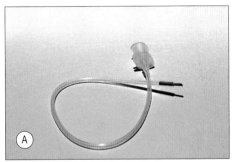

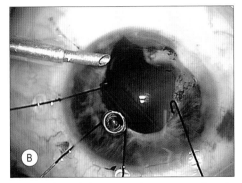

■ **FIGURE 14.3** (**A**) An anterior chamber maintainer. This is put through the cornea via a paracentesis and connected to the irrigation bottle. (**B**) The anterior chamber maintainer in use during an anterior segment reconstruction following trauma.

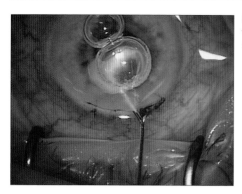

FIGURE 14.4 Triamcinolone being injected into the anterior chamber. This will help visualize vitreous strands beautifully and help in their removal.

injected into the anterior chamber; this can be done with the neat preservative-free preparation (40 mg/ml), but some surgeons prefer to let the particulate drug settle and remove the supernatant before injecting the particles. Either way, the particles stick very well to any vitreous in the anterior segment, and the vitreous can then be visualized easily and thoroughly removed. There are a number of complications of intraocular triamcinolone that need to be considered, not the least of which is glaucoma in a steroid-responder.

A dry surgical sponge is very good at attracting vitreous, and once the anterior vitrectomy is completed, a dry sponge held against the wound and side ports is a good way of ascertaining whether any residual vitreous is attached to the wound. A high cut rate for the vitreous cutter ensures minimal vitreous traction during the vitrectomy, and movements of the cutting device in the eye should be slow and purposeful, avoiding a stirring movement. It is worth preserving the lens capsule as far as possible, as any remaining anterior capsule can be used to support a posterior chamber lens in the sulcus. A slow infusion rate should be used during the vitrectomy to ensure that more vitreous is not forced out of the posterior segment; indeed, some surgeons prefer to perform a dry vitrectomy, with no infusion, for the first part of the procedure, adding slow infusion only once the globe starts to soften.

Vitreous loss during extracapsular surgery

Exactly the same principles apply, but the initial management of any remaining nuclear fragment may be slightly different. If a large proportion of the nucleus remains, it may be possible to use an irrigating vectis (see Fig. 14.5), although care must be taken to avoid putting undue traction on the vitreous during delivery of the nucleus. There is no place in modern surgery for 'sponge and scissors' vitrectomy, as this will cause traction on the vitreous base and may induce a retinal detachment. It is somewhat easier to separate the irrigation and cutter with an extracapsular operation because of the large wound, and again triamcinolone is a very useful adjunct to visualize any remaining

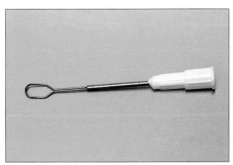

■ **FIGURE 14.5** The irrigating vectis. This is connected to the irrigation bottle and can be used to retrieve a nucleus during extracapsular surgery. Care must be taken not to put traction on the vitreous during this maneuver, and it is sometimes necessary to perform a limited anterior vitrectomy before the nucleus is actually delivered.

vitreous in the anterior segment. The aims of the vitrectomy are to remove vitreous from the anterior segment completely, and prevent any future anteroposterior traction, by removing the anterior third of the vitreous body. If these aims are achieved, excellent results can be obtained and primary lens implantation can still proceed.

POSTOPERATIVE COMPLICATIONS

Endophthalmitis

Endophthalmitis is the most feared of all cataract complications, apart perhaps from a sudden expulsive hemorrhage during extracapsular surgery. Endophthalmitis can be acute or chronic, and the cardinal sign is one of pain. Reduced vision and redness of the eye usually accompany this, and these symptoms should never be ignored. The patient typically presents in the first week after surgery, and early intervention is critical to try to treat these eyes. The use of aqueous povidone iodine 5% preoperatively almost certainly reduces the risk, by virtue of reducing bacterial counts on the ocular surface.[4]

Once the diagnosis is made or suspected, samples from the anterior segment and posterior segment should be taken and subjected to Gram stain microscopy culture and sensitivities. Aqueous biopsy can be carried out at the slit lamp but, as vitreous is also required, both can be sampled perhaps more adequately in the operating theater. A mechanized vitreous cutter is probably the best tool for biopsying the vitreous, and although some authorities advocate a needle tap under local anesthesia, there is the theoretical risk of inducing vitreoretinal traction by doing this. It is likely, however, that the vitreous at this stage is fairly liquefied, which may reduce the risk of this.[5] The Endophthalmitis Vitrectomy Study demonstrated that vitrectomy was beneficial only in eyes with worse than hand movements vision. Antibiotic treatment should be broad-spectrum and intracameral, and commonly used antibiotics are vancomycin 1–2 mg/100 µL plus ceftazidime 2.25 mg/100 µL; amikacin can be used instead of ceftazidime in the dose of 400 mg/100 µL. Other agents should be considered if unusual organisms are suspected. For example, amphotericin B can be used for fungal infection.

The use of oral antibiotic, topical antibiotic, and oral steroid therapy has not been shown to convincingly alter the course of events, so if a patient fails to respond within 2 or 3 days to the intraocular antibiotics, further doses should be given by that route. It is common though to administer topical antibiotics at the same time, as these can be continued postoperatively for a number of weeks to ensure that any surface organisms are eliminated.

If an outbreak of infectious endophthalmitis occurs, systems should be in place to analyze the potential causes.[6]

Chronic endophthalmitis

This is defined as starting 6 weeks or more after surgery, and the most common organism causing the syndrome is *Propionibacterium acnes*. The main features are a low-grade infection with keratic precipitates and plaque-like deposits on the posterior capsule, which harbor the organisms. Despite intravitreal antibiotics, these cases can become very chronic, and sometimes physical removal of the lens capsule is necessary to cure the condition.

Chronic cystoid macular edema

Subclinical macular edema is reported to be relatively common, but it is usually self-limiting. Undoubtedly, chronic uveitis or vitreomacular traction can exacerbate the condition. Certainly, vitreous loss at surgery, wherein residual vitreous is attached to the wound, can induce the condition; it is known then as the Irvine–Gass syndrome. Chronic cystoid macular edema is most easily picked up nowadays by optical coherence tomography (OCT) scanning, as shown in Figure 14.6. Fluorescein angiography is also useful, but OCT is much less invasive and gives adequate information. Causes should be sought, such as vitreous incarceration in the cataract wound, or chronic inflammation. Oral acetazolamide can be very useful in treating cystoid macular edema, and the condition can be surprisingly dependent on a small dose of acetazolamide to keep it under control. If this is the case, then it is possible that vitreous traction exists, and if such traction is visible, then it is advisable to carry out a vitrectomy to relieve the traction, to reduce the patient's dependence on acetazolamide.

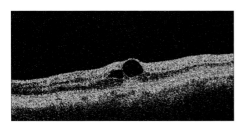

■ **FIGURE 14.6** An optical coherence tomography scan showing cystoid macular edema, following cataract surgery, often due to persistent anteroposterior vitreoretinal traction from vitreous caught in the wound (the Irvine–Gass syndrome).

Posterior capsular opacification

This causes a gradual but significant drop in visual acuity and can occur quite slowly, sometimes several years after the surgery. Preventive measures include cortical cleavage hydrodissection, careful soft lens matter removal, and removal of residual lens epithelial cells, as well as central placement of the implant in the bag with the rim of anterior capsule overlapping the edge of the implant. Other factors, such as implant design and material, may be important.[7]

Yttrium–aluminum–garnet (YAG) laser capsulotomy can effectively treat the condition by opening the capsule and clearing the visual axis. Although there are reports of retinal detachment associated with YAG laser capsulotomy, in our unit a retrospective study over 10 years has demonstrated no retinal detachments in patients in whom the energy per pulse of capsulotomy was kept below 1.2 mJ. This may be because the induced shock with each pulse on the capsule, and therefore the zonules, is much less, and therefore the risk of post-oral breaks is reduced. This remains to be ratified experimentally, but certainly clinically seems to be important.

Refractive surprises

Careful biometry usually produces excellent optical results, but refractive surprises can occur for a number of reasons. This can lead to visual discomfort, especially if the two eyes are significantly anisometropic. A number of methods to overcome this can be tried, including spectacles, contact lenses, and ultimately implant exchange or implant piggybacking. Some implants fibrose reasonably rapidly into the capsular bag and are difficult to remove. Others can easily be removed even years after surgery. Acrysof lenses (Alcon) are easily removed, whereas AMO CEE-ON Edge lenses tend to stick firmly in the capsular bag because of the shape of the shoulder of the haptic. In cases where the lenses are easily removed, they can be replaced by an appropriate-strength implant. Where a lens is difficult to remove, then a piggyback might be a better option, and the appropriate strength can be implanted on top of the existing implant, according to the formula shown in Table 14.1. Some examples:

- Residual error + 3.0 diopters: corrective piggyback lens = 3 × 1.5 = 4.5 diopters.
- Residual error –4.0 diopters: Corrective piggyback lens = –4 × 1 = –4 diopters.

TABLE 14.1 Formulae for calculating strength of 'piggyback' lens

Residual error	Hypermetropic	Myopic
Corrective additional lens	Error × 1.5	Error × 1

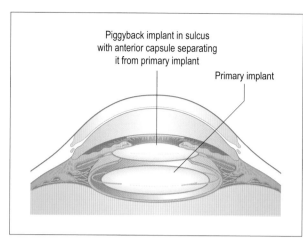

Piggyback implant in sulcus
with anterior capsule separating
it from primary implant

Primary implant

■ **FIGURE 14.7** Piggyback intraocular lens implantation to correct refractive surprises. The correct position for a piggyback lens, which is placed in the ciliary sulcus with the leaves of the anterior capsule between it and the primary posterior chamber lens. This prevents lens epithelial cell growth at the lens interface.

Figure 14.7 shows a piggyback implant and the importance of placing the piggyback lens outside the capsular bag and in the sulcus, so that the anterior capsular rim lies between the two lens optics. This seems to prevent growth of lens epithelial cells between the implants.

REFERENCES

1. Gillow JT, Aggarwal RK, Kirkby GR. Ocular perforation during peribulbar anaesthesia. Eye 1996; 10(part 5):533–536.
2. Lewis H, Blumenkranz NS, Chang S. Treatment of dislocated crystalline lens and retinal detachment with perfluorocarbon liquids. Retina 1992; 12:299–304.
3. Singh DV, Pal N, Sharma YR, et al. Intracameral triamcinolone helps to visualise and remove the vitreous body in anterior chamber in cataract surgery. Am J Ophthalmol 2005; 139(4):756.
4. Apt L, Isenberg SJ, Yoshimori R, et al. Chemical preparation of the eye in ophthalmic surgery: part III. Effect of povidone–iodine on the conjunctiva. Arch Ophthalmol 1984; 102:728–729.
5. Endophthalmitis Vitrectomy Study Group. Results of the endophthalmitis vitrectomy study. A randomised trial of immediate vitrectomy and of intravenous antibiotics for the treatment of post-operative bacterial endophthalmitis. Arch Ophthalmol 1995; 113:1479–1496.
6. Rogers NK, Fox PD, Noble BA, et al. Aggressive management of an epidemic of chronic pseudophakic endophthalmitis: results and literature survey. Br J Ophthalmol 1994; 78(2):115–119.
7. Born CP, Ryan DK. Effect of intraocular lens optic design on posterior capsular opacification. J Cataract Refract Surg 1990; 16:188–192.

15 Lens exchange (including refractive lens exchange)

Despite advances in biometric techniques and surgical planning, unacceptable refractive error, or anisometropia, still occurs in a small proportion of patients. Johansson states that 1% of patients with significant anisometropia did not report any binocularity problems.[1] However, these situations do occur. Evidence is also accruing for certain types of implants giving rise to dysphotopsia; more can be read on this in Chapter 16 (*Wavefront aberrometry and cataract surgery*).

Exchanging an intraocular lens implant for another should never be taken lightly, as the possible complications are very similar to those of the original cataract surgery, with the exception of course of the possibility of a dropped nucleus. However, infection, retinal detachment, and other sight-threatening conditions can still occur, and there is no guarantee that the new desired refractive state will be achieved. On the occasions when lens exchange does become necessary, careful examination of the lens–capsular bag complex should be made to ascertain the degree of in the bag placement and whether this is present through 360°. It is not uncommon for one leaf of the anterior capsule to position itself behind the back of the implant against the posterior capsule and fuse solidly to the posterior capsule. This occurs especially if the original capsulorrhexis was larger than the diameter of the implant. Certain types of implant seem to stick fast in the capsular bag; an example of this is the AMO CEE-ON lens, which, because of the angulated shoulder of the haptic as it comes out of the optic, can be extremely difficult to remove. On the other hand Acrysof (Alcon, Fort Worth, Texas) lenses are easily removed even a year or two after surgery. If at surgery the implant is found to be stuck solidly in the capsular bag, it is probably safer to use a piggyback implant, and the formula for calculating which strength of piggyback implant to use and the way in which the implant is positioned with respect to the primary implant are discussed in Chapter 14 (*Management of complications*).

IMPLANT RETRIEVAL

The three main methods of implant retrieval are first to cut it in some way (Fig. 15.1) and remove it from the eye; second, to refold it within the eye; and third, to create a large 7-mm scleral tunnel and remove the lens intact through this opening. Each of these will be considered in turn.

Cutting the lens

The first maneuver with any of the procedures to remove the lens is to remove the intraocular lens from the capsular bag. This can be done with a combination of viscodissection and gentle manipulation with a cyclodialysis spatula or something similar. Figure 15.2 shows a tripod lens being flip-flopped out of the capsular bag, and Figure 15.3 shows a three-piece lens having just been dialed out of the bag. It takes a reasonable amount of force to cut through a folding intraocular lens, and various implements have been designed

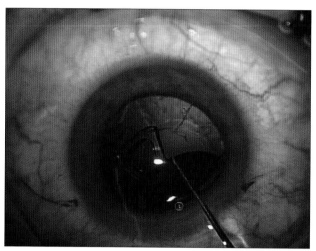

■ **FIGURE 15.2** A tripod lens having one of its plate haptics flip-flopped out of the capsular bag.

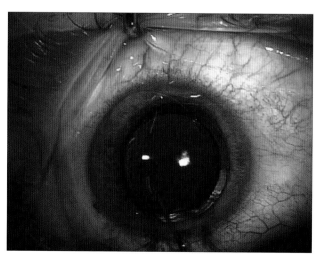

■ **FIGURE 15.3** An Acrysof lens being dialed out of the capsular bag. This remains possible even 12 months after the surgery.

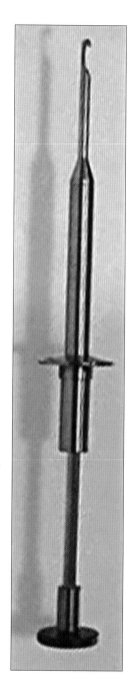

■ **FIGURE 15.1** The intraocular lens cutter from John Weiss.

to do this. Figure 15.4 shows a specially designed pair of scissors being used to cut through the lens; if this method is used, it must be remembered that the edge of the lens must be stabilized to prevent it from flipping up against the endothelium as the jaws of the scissors close. It is necessary to cut through only three-quarters of the diameter of the lens, as it can then be rotated out of the eye after the leading edge of the cut segment is delivered out of the wound; the lens is rotated through 360° to deliver it from the eye. Figure 15.5A shows the tip of a device designed by John Weiss called a lens cutter. The tip of this device has a sliding razor blade that is operated by a plunger under the surgeon's thumb. Figure 15.5B shows a lens in the process of being cut in half with this device, and Figure 15.6 a fragment being delivered from the eye.

Refolding the lens

Again, the lens is dislocated from the capsular bag and copious amounts of viscoelastic placed in the anterior chamber above and below the implant. A stout cylindric metal instrument is placed below the lens through the main wound and positioned exactly under its maximum diameter. The forceps that are used to deliver the lens into the eye are then placed through the main wound, and the lens is folded over the cylindric metal instrument, such as a dialer, which is carefully removed before the lens is completely folded. The lens can then be rotated through 90° and delivered out of the same wound through which it was inserted. This refolding technique should be carried out slowly to ensure that the haptics do not snag the posterior capsule as the lens is refolded. It must be remembered that the wound must be opened to the size through which a folded lens can be delivered, and this is usually larger than the original size of the wound made for admitting the phacoemulsification

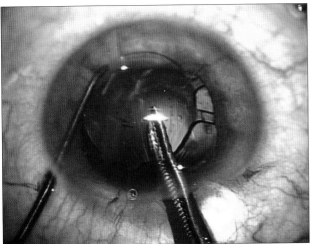

■ **FIGURE 15.4** Specialized scissors being used to cut an intraocular lens before removal from the anterior chamber.

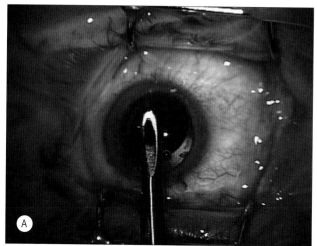

A

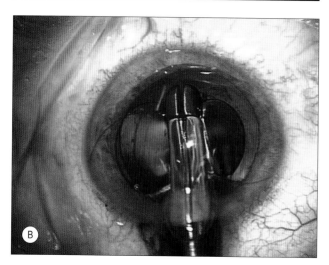

B

FIGURE 15.5 (**A**) Detail of the tip of the lens cutter from John Weiss. (**B**) The cutter in use. As the instrument's plunger is pressed, a blade advances through the implant, completely bisecting it.

probe. Manufacturers are often optimistic in quoting the size of wound through which a lens can be placed, and it is better to make this wound a little larger, and close it with a suture afterward if necessary, than to try to forcefully deliver the lens through a wound that is too small.

Scleral tunnel

The conjunctivum is opened and a 6- to 7-mm scleral wound is fashioned 2 mm from the limbus. This is tunneled forward into the anterior chamber after initial downward dissection and the implant, which has been dislocated from the capsular bag, can be delivered whole through this wound. Although it is a large wound, because it is so posterior it usually induces very little astigmatism and can be closed with nylon sutures and recovered by conjunctiva. Although employing a larger wound, this technique is probably the safest from the point of view of preserving endothelial cells.

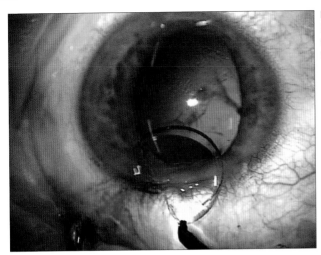

■ **FIGURE 15.6** Removal of a lens segment after being cut with the lens cutter from John Weiss.

Figure 15.7A shows a one-piece lens being removed via a scleral wound and Figure 15.7B the replacement lens in situ.

INSERTING THE NEW IMPLANT

The new implant is inserted in the normal way with either folding forceps or an injector cartridge, or placed unfolded through a scleral wound if that is the method that has been employed to remove the old implant. Figure 15.8 shows a Tecnis Z9000 lens being reinserted into the capsular bag following removal of a lens causing severe dysphotopsia (see Ch. 16, *Wavefront aberrometry and cataract surgery*). The corneal wound, if it has been made, is hydrated after removal of the viscoelastic. If the new lens cannot be placed within the capsular bag in the same position as the old one, recalculation of the biometry should be undertaken to allow for slight forward displacement of the lens if it is to sit in the ciliary sulcus. Careful initial calculations must be made to take account of probable differences in the A constant of the lens to be removed and the new one to be implanted.

REFRACTIVE LENS EXCHANGE

The technique of refractive lens exchange is becoming increasingly popular, partly because laser refractive surgery is not suitable for all refractive errors and partly because, with the development of multifocal implants, the treatment of presbyopia has become a reality. Although modern refractive lens exchange usually offers safe visual rehabilitation, according to patients' needs, virtually all the specific complications of cataract surgery are possible and should be discussed with patients who are contemplating this procedure. There are also more specific complications relating to the nature and type of surgery, and their management will be discussed later.

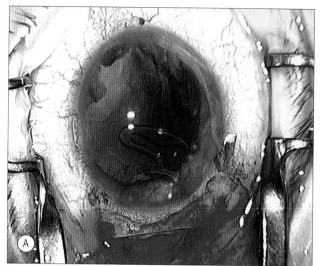

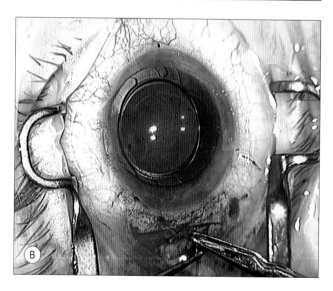

■ **FIGURE 15.7** (**A**) Removal of an intact lens implant via a 6-mm scleral tunnel. Although a large wound, it is sufficiently posterior to remain astigmatically neutral. (**B**) The new lens in place after being easily implanted through the scleral tunnel.

Indications

High hypermetropia and high myopia

These conditions are often not treatable with excimer laser because of the relative depth of ablation required for myopia, or the lack of consistently good results for high hypermetropes. These patients often have a much better quality of vision with contact lenses and certainly, if they become intolerant of lenses, refractive lens exchange can offer a good alternative. Many patients also complain of the weight and cost of their spectacles, and although this is a relative indication it is important to some patients.

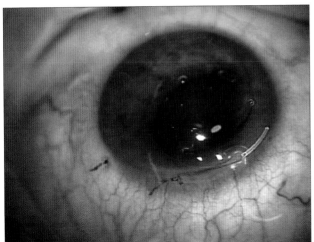

■ **FIGURE 15.8** A Tecnis Z9000 being implanted to replace the explanted spherical lens that was associated with dysphotopsias caused by spherical aberration.

Presbyopia

One of the consequences of the ever-expanding crystalline lens, presbyopia is deemed by some to be a disease process and by others simply an aging phenomenon. Either way, if a patient has very early cataract and is contemplating a refractive procedure, then refractive lens exchange would seem logical rather than considering laser corneal refractive surgery and subsequent cataract surgery, with all the attendant difficulties that laser refractive surgery produces in calculating optimal lens implant strength. Some patients simply wish to dispense with the need for glasses for reading once they are presbyopic, and surgery for this reason is gaining popularity because of the use of multifocal implants, allowing good uncorrected distance and near vision. However, it must be remembered that most studies still show a need for glasses wear, for some of the time, in a proportion of patients.[2]

Table 15.1 shows the design features of various modern multifocal implants in use today. Various studies have compared the use of different multifocal lens designs with monofocal lenses,[3,4] and some of the potential problems, such as reduction in contrast sensitivity and glare, have also been addressed looking at different types of implant.[5] These issues must be addressed before implanting such lenses into patients, as the relative advantage of unaided reading vision must be weighed against the potential loss of contrast at distance and under mesopic conditions. The most modern multifocal lenses combine an aspheric surface with a diffractive multifocal element, and these are showing promise in clinical trials.

TABLE 15.1 Comparison of three multifocal intraocular implants

Lens type	Design	Material	Refractive component	Size	Filter
AMO Array	Zonal progressive with refractive zones on anterior surface. Three-piece design with square edge.	Silicone	Zones 1, 3, and 5 are distance-dominant, zones 2 and 4 near-dominant	6-mm optic, 13-mm overall diameter.	Ultraviolet
Alcon ReStore	Apodized refractive zone (3.6 mm) providing two foci; surrounded by purely refractive outer zone. One-piece design with square edge.	Hydrophobic acrylic (Acrysof)	Twelve-zone central diffractive, apodized zone; surrounding 2.4-mm refractive zone	6-mm optic, 13-mm overall diameter.	Ultraviolet and blue light
AMO ReZoom	Five-zone, three-piece design with square edge.	Second-generation silicone/acrylic	Five zones giving distance-dominant central zone—more active with small pupil in photopic conditions	6-mm optic, 13-mm overall diameter.	Ultraviolet

IMPLANTATION OF MULTIFOCAL LENS

A study by Packer has shown that for optimal performance these lenses must suffer no more than 7° of tilt and 0.4 mm of decentration, although revision of these figures recently has shown that the lenses can tolerate more decentration and more tilt before they become optically compromised. The capsulorrhexis must be central, round, and smaller than the diameter of the optic, as it is generally considered that a capsulorrhexis of between 4 and 5 mm is optimal. This is for two reasons. First, it allows full use of the multizone components of these lenses, as anterior capsular opacification will obscure the more peripheral components, and if it is less than 4 mm this will have a deleterious effect on the optics. Additionally, the advent of posterior capsular opacification will obviously cause optical problems, and the incidence of this is lessened if the edge of the capsulorrhexis overlies the anterior surface of the optic. Figure 15.9 shows an implant with one edge of the anterior capsular rim being larger than the implant optic. In this area, lens epithelial cells have grown along the posterior capsule and have caused opacification. In the area where anterior capsule overlies the optic edge, no such ingrowth has occurred. If the capsulorrhexis is smaller than 4 mm, then capsular phimosis can ensue; this can be difficult to deal with surgically and will negate some of the optical advantages of these multifocal designs.

Careful biometry is mandatory, as significant deviation from emmetropia will require either additional surgical procedures or wearing of two pairs of glasses for optimal vision at distance and near. Either partial coherence interferometry (IOL Master, Carl Zeiss Meditec, Dublin, California) or immersion ultrasound should be used, as applanation biometry is too prone to inaccuracies to allow repeatable results.

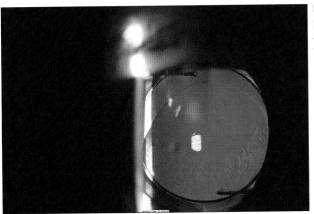

■ **FIGURE 15.9** Partial posterior capsule opacification allowed by non-overlapping of the anterior capsular edge inferiorly on the optic.

ACCOMMODATIVE INTRAOCULAR LENS IMPLANTATION

A number of new lens designs are on trial, and some seem to give reasonable results under trial conditions.[6] Because these lenses tend not to use multifocal designs but rather depend on vitreous pressure generating forward movement of the implant with accommodative effort, they tend to give superior contrast sensitivity results to the multifocal lenses. The amplitude of accommodation may be smaller than that required in a proportion of patients, therefore requiring additional correction for near, especially under mesopic conditions. A particular complication of these lenses is their dislocation out of the capsular bag with accommo-dative effort, following which they must be replaced to ensure continued functional accommodation.

OTHER DEVELOPMENTS

The Calhoun light-adjustable lens is an exciting develop-ment that in theory allows the adjustment of the intra-ocular lens power some days after implantation by exposure to ultraviolet light. In theory, this would allow crystalline lens removal, light-adjustable lens implantation followed by wavefront assessment of the residual total aberrations, and final adjustment of the intraocular implant using ultra-violet light. Trials of this lens are under way, but it will still provide monofocal correction unless a way can be found to cause multifocal change of the implant subsequent to surgery.

INJECTABLE VISCOPOLYMERS

Experiments in primates have shown that if the capsular bag is emptied through a 1-mm capsulorrhexis and residual lens epithelial cells are removed with a cytotoxic agent, the lens bag can be reinflated with one of a number of viscopolymers and some degree of accommodation can be achieved. Tech-niques such as this seem attractive, but it is as yet un-known whether they will be functionally adequate in the aging eye, where ciliary body function is perhaps reduced. Certainly, for younger patients it may be the way forward.

SUMMARY

The development of refractive lens exchange has been revolutionized by the development of multifocal implants, and this development continues. For cataract patients, these implants offer some advantages, although the issues of loss of contrast sensitivity and glare and haloes must be dis-cussed. For myopic and presbyopic patients who do not have cataract, this surgery offers advantageous change to their visual status, but clear discussions about potential com-plications must be undertaken so that patients are aware of the risks, however small, to their otherwise healthy eyes.

REFERENCES

1. Johansson P. Resulting refraction after same day bilateral phacoemulsification. J Cataract Refract Surg 2004; 30(6):1326–1334.
2. US Food and Drug Administration. Summary of safety and effectiveness data. Online. Available: http://www.fda.gov/cdrh/pdf4/p040020b.pdf
3. Steinert RF, Post CT, Brint SF, et al. A progressive, randomized, double-masked comparison of a zonal-progressive multifocal intraocular lens and a monofocal intraocular lens. Ophthalmology 1992; 99:853–836.
4. Brydon KW, Tokarewicz AC, Nichols BD. AMO Array multifocal lens versus monofocal correction in cataract surgery. J Cataract Refract Surg 2000; 26:96–100.
5. Pieh S, Weghaupt H, Skorpik C. Contrast sensitivity and glare disability with diffractive and refractive multifocal intraocular lenses. J Cataract Refract Surg 1998; 24:659–662.
6. Cumming JS, Colvard DM, Dell SJ, et al. Clinical evaluation of the Crystalens AT-45 accommodating intraocular lens: results of the US Food and Drug Administration clinical trial. J Cataract Refract Surg 2006; 32(5):812–825.

16 Wavefront aberrometry and cataract surgery

WAVEFRONT ABERROMETRY

This technique, which is increasingly employed in laser refractive surgery to determine preoperative aberrations produced by the eye's optical system, is becoming better utilized in the pre- and postoperative assessment of cataract patients. Various aberrometers exist. Figure 16.1 shows the Bausch & Lomb wavefront analyzer. The principle of these machines is that they emit a pulse of infrared light into the eye, which is reflected by the retina. As the resulting wavefront is emitted back out of the eye through the eye's various optical media, it is changed, or aberrated, by the media through which it passes. Using an array of lenslets, the aberrometer measures the deviation from an ideal wavefront, produced by the eye's optics, and shows an aberrometry map of these deviations produced by the eye under examination. The map so produced gives the total aberrations produced by the eye; it does not single out a particular optical structure, such as the lens or the cornea, but shows a combined effect of all the optical structures.

The Bausch & Lomb aberrometer uses Zernike polynomials to interpret the wavefront and gives second-, third-, fourth-, and fifth-order aberrations arising from the eye. Table 16.1 defines the different higher-order aberrations. Figure 16.2 shows a typical aberrometry map produced in a preoperative patient. Sachdev et al. in New Zealand have performed aberrometry on preoperative patients. Their findings indicate that nuclear cataract seems to induce negative fourth-order spherical aberration, while cortical cataracts are associated with coma.[1] In Figure 16.2, the

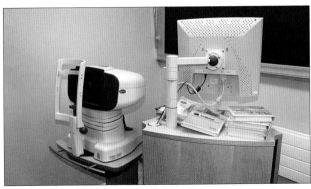

FIGURE 16.1 The Bausch & Lomb Zywave aberrometer.

TABLE 16.1 Definitions of higher-order aberrations

Order	Definition
First	Tilt along x- and y-axes
Second	Spherical refractive error (defocus) and astigmatism
Third	Coma and trefoil
Fourth	Spherical aberration, secondary astigmatism, and tetrafoil
Fifth	Secondary coma and secondary trefoil and pentafoil

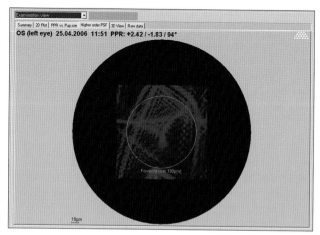

FIGURE 16.2 A typical wavefront map of a highly aberrated eye. This shows the point spread function of light emitted from the eye.

patient had a large amount of spherical aberration arising from a mainly nuclear cataract, and these aberrations can induce visual disturbance that is separate to the effect on clarity that the cataract has. Compare this with Figure 16.3, which shows perfect unaberrated wavefront.

The importance of wavefront analysis has come to light recently with the advent of aspheric intraocular lens, whose front surface has been made prolate as opposed to oblate. This means that the radius of curvature of the anterior surface of the lens is modified to be less curved at the edges than it is in the middle. This technology has been employed in camera lenses for many years and results in higher contrast and sharper images. The first intraocular lens to be introduced with this technology was the Tecnis Z9000, now marketed by AMO, and this has been shown in a number of studies to give better contrast under mesopic conditions.[2] Wavefront has also been able to explain a number of cases of dysphotopsia, in which patients' symptoms are very difficult to quantify other than by wavefront aberrometry. An example of such a case follows.

A 63-year-old woman was referred from another unit a year after uneventful cataract surgery. Although her visual acuity was 20/20 (6/6) unaided, she complained of glare,

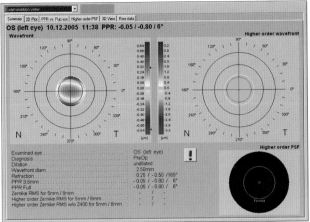

■ **FIGURE 16.3** A perfect wavefront. As can be seen, the blue and mauve circles in the map at bottom right are not aberrated at all and have a non-altered point spread function. The aberration map (top right) is absolutely uniform.

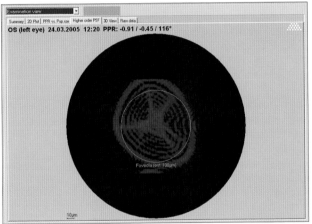

■ **FIGURE 16.4** Point spread function map of a 63-year-old woman's eye after spherical lens implantation.

reflections, and other symptoms difficult to describe. She underwent wavefront aberrometry and Figure 16.4 shows the resultant aberration map. The software on the Bausch & Lomb machine allows different higher-order aberrations to be switched on and off to anticipate which of these aberrations is causing the symptoms. Figure 16.5 shows the Zernike polynomial chart superimposed on the wavefront in Figure 16.4. As can be seen, the central spherical aberration icon has been switched off, as denoted by the red cross through the icon.

The resultant map shown in Figure 16.5 shows a dramatic decrease in the aberrations, thus indicating that the spherical aberration was mainly responsible for the symptoms she was experiencing. She was offered a lens exchange for an aspheric monofocal implant, and following this her dysphotopsia symptoms disappeared.

The reason that this sort of dysphotopsia occurs is a mismatch between the spherical aberration of the cornea and the lens. In young people, the corneal aberration is positive

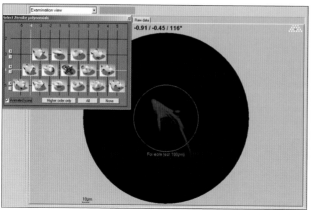

FIGURE 16.5 The same 63-year-old patient's eye with the software switching off of the spherical aberration, showing a large improvement in the point spread function map.

in its dimension, while that of the young crystalline lens is negative. The two virtually cancel one another out to ensure sharp vision. As the crystalline lens ages and thickens, the spherical aberration changes to positive and adds to that of the cornea. When cataract surgery is performed, a normal spherical intraocular lens will not provide any balancing effect of the positive corneal spherical aberration, and indeed adds to it, and it is this additional positive spherical aberration that is almost certainly responsible for a proportion of the dysphotopsias reported postoperatively. In my experience, the dysphotopsia is more often reported in patients in the 50- to 60-year age group. By introducing an intraocular lens with a negative overall spherical aberration, this will cancel out the corneal positive spherical aberration and give a better quality of vision.

Two further types of aspheric implant are now available. The IQ (Alcon, Fort Worth, Texas) and the SofPort (Bausch & Lomb, Rochester, New York), although similar in design to the Tecnis, both introduce different amounts of correction of spherical aberration. Tecnis Z9000 has a lens spherical aberration of $-0.27\,\mu m$, giving a residual spherical aberration of zero. The Acrysof IQ has a lens spherical aberration of $-0.2\,\mu m$ and an average residual spherical aberration of $0.1\,\mu m$. The SofPort AO lens has a zero lens spherical aberration and an average residual spherical aberration of $+0.28\,\mu m$. Each company presents a slightly different argument for the residual spherical aberration. The argument behind leaving an average positive spherical aberration with the latter two lenses is that it increases depth of focus, while the argument for the Tecnis Z9000 is that with a zero residual spherical aberration contrast sensitivity in mesopic conditions is improved due to their being no residual aberration. The calculations for residual spherical aberration for the Acrysof IQ and SofPort AO were both made on larger numbers of corneae than the original Tecnis Z9000 estimations.

More work needs to be done on residual spherical aberration in different age groups, as is illustrated by the following case.

An 18-year-old woman presented with a posterior subcapsular cataract in one eye. She had a past ophthalmic history of a sphenoid ridge meningioma, for which she underwent localized radiotherapy some years previously. She underwent uneventful cataract surgery and had a Tecnis Z9000 lens implanted in her left eye (this surgery was carried out when it was the only aspheric lens available); the residual wavefront map is shown in Figure 16.6. She has a little persistent spherical aberration following the surgery, probably because of her young age and the fact that the Tecnis has left her with too much residual negative spherical aberration. Figure 16.7 shows the spherical aberration switched off by the software in the Zywave machine. She may have benefited more from one of the newer lenses with less negative spherical aberration. However, she also has a lot of trouble with the lack of reading addition and is now

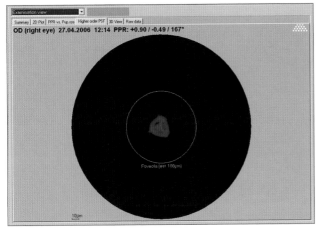

■ **FIGURE 16.6** The residual wavefront map after implantation of a Tecnis Z9000 in an 18-year-old woman.

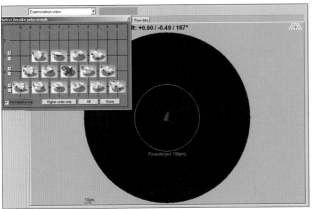

■ **FIGURE 16.7** The residual wavefront point spread function of the 18-year-old patient's eye after switching off the spherical aberration. She may have benefited more from a less corrected lens, i.e. one with less negative spherical aberration.

contemplating having a lens exchange for a multifocal implant to make reading easier.

Figure 16.8 shows the postoperative result in a 70-year-old male patient after the implantation of an Acrysof IQ aspheric lens. This lens also incorporates Alcon's yellow chromophore filter and is a hydrophobic acrylic one-piece implant. Figure 16.9 shows the implant at the end of surgery. Figure 16.10 demonstrates that the aberration map does not change when the spherical aberration is turned off, indicating that the residual aberrations are not due to spherical aberration. Figure 16.11 demonstrates that turning off the lower-order aberrations results in a significantly improved aberration map.

Another measurement provided by the wavefront aberrometry apparatus is the predicted phoropter refraction, wherein the refraction is predicted at different pupil sizes and represented graphically. Figure 16.12 shows a map for

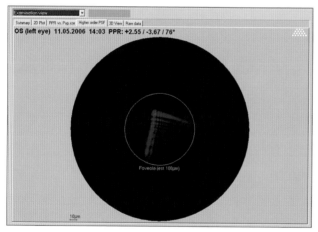

■ **FIGURE 16.8** Postoperative point spread function map of an eye implanted with the Alcon IQ aspheric lens.

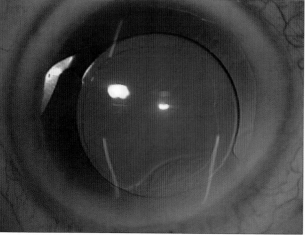

■ **FIGURE 16.9** The Alcon IQ aspheric lens at the end of the phacoemulsification procedure.

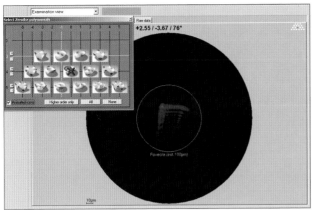

■ **FIGURE 16.10** The same map as in Figure 16.8 with the spherical aberration turned off. This shows that negligible spherical aberration is present postoperatively.

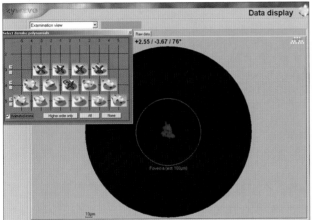

■ **FIGURE 16.11** Turning off the lower-order aberrations (focus and astigmatism) improves the point spread function map from Figures 16.8 and 16.10. This demonstrates that the residual aberration is a small amount of defocus and not spherical aberration.

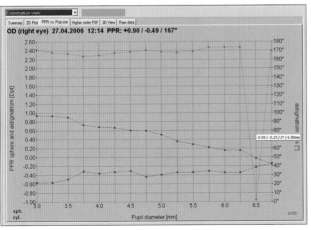

■ **FIGURE 16.12** The predicted phoropter refraction at different pupil sizes from the 18-year-old patient's eye. This shows significant myopic shift with larger pupil sizes.

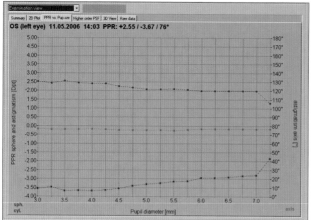

FIGURE 16.13 Phoropter refraction of the Alcon IQ lens. This shows no myopic shift with an increase in pupil size from 3 to 7 mm.

the 18-year-old patient who had a Tecnis Z9000 lens; it clearly shows that at pupil sizes of above 4 mm the blue line on the graph indicates the spherical change changes by about a diopter. This indicates that her vision under mesopic conditions will almost certainly be more blurred due to pupil enlargement–induced myopic shift. Figure 16.13 shows the same type of chart for the 70-year-old with an IQ lens, showing very little shift in spherical correction over pupil enlargement from 3 to 7 mm.

This function of predictive phoropter refraction can be a very useful tool in analyzing some symptomatology for patients with dysphotopsia. Indeed, a paper by McDonald et al. demonstrates the effect of brimonidine tartrate 0.2% on pupil size;[3] if such myopic shift under mesopic conditions does occur, then it is worth trying this drug to reduce nighttime dysphotopsia.

Wavefront technology is very useful in analyzing the total aberrations of the eye as an optical system, and software will soon be available that will enable aberrations from the cornea to be differentiated from those of the lens. This will be incredibly useful for analyzing and interpreting data arising from the implantation of new styles of aspheric, multifocal, and accommodative implants.

REFERENCES

1. Sachdev N, Ormonde SE, Sherwin T, et al. Higher-order aberrations of lenticular opacities. J Cataract Refract Surg 2004; 30(8):1642–1648.
2. Packer M, Fine IH, Hoffman RS, et al. Initial clinical experience with an anterior surface modified prolate intraocular lens. J Refract Surg 2002; 18:692–696.
3. McDonald JE, El-Moatassem Kotb AM, Decker BB. Effect of brimonidine tartrate ophthalmic solution 0.2% on pupil size in normal eyes under different luminescence conditions. J Cataract Refract Surg 2001; 27:560–564.

Index